W9-DFH-612

# THE HOSPICE MOVEMENT

*Easing Death's Pains*

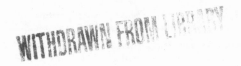
WITHDRAWN FROM LIBRARY

# SOCIAL MOVEMENTS PAST AND PRESENT

## Irwin T. Sanders, Editor

MONTGOMERY COLLEGE
ROCKVILLE CAMPUS LIBRARY
ROCKVILLE, MARYLAND

# THE HOSPICE MOVEMENT

## *Easing Death's Pains*

*Cathy Siebold*

Twayne Publishers • New York

Maxwell Macmillan Canada • Toronto

Maxwell Macmillan International • New York   Oxford   Singapore   Sydney

OCT 2 6 1993

AA 3 P329

*The Hospice Movement: Easing Death's Pains*
by Cathy Siebold

Copyright 1992 by Twayne Publishers

All rights reserved. No part of this book may be reproduced or transmitted in any form or by any means, electronic or mechanical, including photocopying, recording, or by any information storage and retrieval system, without permission in writing from the Publisher.

Twayne Publishers
Macmillan Publishing Company
866 Third Avenue
New York, New York  10022

Maxwell Macmillan Canada, Inc.
1200 Eglinton Avenue East
Suite 200
Don Mills, Ontario  M3C 3N1

Macmillan Publishing Company is a part of the Maxwell Communication Group of Companies.

**Library of Congress Cataloging-in-Publication Data**
Siebold, Cathy.
The hospice movement : easing death's pains / Cathy Siebold.
    p.  cm. — (Social movements past and present)
    Includes bibliographical references and index.
    ISBN 0-8057-3867-3 (cloth). — ISBN 0-8057-3868-1 (pbk.)
    1. Hospice care—History.  I. Title.  II. Series.
        R726.8.S54  1992
362.1'75—dc20                                           92-18052
                                                              CIP

The paper used in this publication meets the minimum requirements of American National Standard for Information Sciences—Permanence of Paper for Printed Library Materials, ANSI Z39.48-1984.

10 9 8 7 6 5 4 3 2 1 (alk. paper)

10 9 8 7 6 5 4 3 2 1 (pbk.: alk. paper)

Printed in the United States of America.

# Contents

# Preface

The word *hospice* has different meanings. During medieval times, hospices were institutions that provided refuge for the sick or travel weary. More recently, *hospice* has come to connote a concept of care aimed at reducing the spiritual, emotional, and physical discomfort accompanying a terminal illness that can be provided anywhere. This concept was little known to traditional health care providers until 1971, when Hospice, Inc., the first modern American hospice program, began providing home care services. This relatively unconventional concept of care has since become part of mainstream medicine, a rare event in a conservative industry.

U.S. hospice programs experienced their greatest period of growth in the 1980s, increasing from about 200 programs in 1980 to 1,500 by 1985. This proliferation resulted from a number of factors, including the ability of supporters to promote the concept and the introduction of legislation instituting insurance reimbursement for hospice services. Despite widespread availability, hospice care remains relatively unknown by the public, and those who are familiar with it are often unaware of the myriad differences in program types.

My experience with hospice care began in the late 1960s, when as a volunteer for a visiting nurse service I was exposed to the idea that dying people need a special kind of care and that the hospital is not the appropriate place for them to spend their last days. Hospices were then "special places" where terminally ill people could receive holistic care and where families could participate in the process. I was intrigued and enthusiastic about this new service. Years later, in the early 1980s, I had the opportunity to work in a hospice program and found that hospice care had changed considerably. My desire to better understand the changes I observed sparked my interest in researching the history of hospice care. My findings are described in this book.

# Acknowledgments

Throughout the process of studying and writing about the evolution of hospice care, I have been assisted by a number of people. Some have shared their experience and knowledge of hospice care, and others have instructed me in the intricacies of writing, thus facilitating the completion of this project.

Numerous individuals who participated in the death with dignity or hospice movement allowed me to interview them. In particular I would like to thank Jean Benoliel, Zelda Foster, Patrice O'Connor, Elizabeth Pritchard, and Carlton Sweetser. Their insights into the hospice movement's early history and the access they gave me to original documents helped me to formulate a comprehensive perspective on the movement's development.

This book is the culmination of several years of research, which first began when I was a doctoral student. I would like to thank Joel Sacks and Norman Linzer at the Wurzweiler School of Social Work in New York, who encouraged and assisted my initial research efforts. In preparing the manuscript I was assisted by Frank Clemente and Darrell Steffensmeier at Penn State University and Bonnie Lazar at the University of Southern Maine. All in different ways gave their advice and support in pursuing and completing the writing of a book.

I am particularly indebted to Irwin Sanders, editor of Twayne's Social Movements Series, for his careful and patient reading and rereading of this manuscript. John Martin, Carol Chin, and India Koopman, editors at Twayne Publishers, also played a part in this process, as did Wendy Bessey, my research assistant, and Mary Flink, who provided secretarial support.

*Chapter 1*

# An Introduction to the Hospice Movement

In 1967 a group of health care professionals gathered to talk about the way that dying people were treated in our culture. This meeting in Connecticut by the Yale Study Group represented the beginning of a social movement that would result in a nationwide network of hospice programs. People came to talk, even gripe, about the way terminally ill patients received aggressive treatments until they died. Such practices seemed to benefit the hospital staff rather than the patient. As one observer noted, "Nobody dies in this country without being cured."

The Yale Study Group's interest in discussing, studying, and changing the way that dying patients and their families were treated resulted in the establishment of the first modern American hospice program and the Hospice National Advisory Council. Moreover, these activities encouraged the formation of other groups across the country whose aim was to improve conditions for dying people by starting hospices.

## A Definition of *Hospice*

Defining the term *hospice* is a difficult task because of the way hospice care evolved in America. Contemporary hospice programs are places or methods of care for dying patients, and the services they offer vary based on the predilection of the group establishing the program. The theme that unifies all hospice providers is their desire to provide some form of

1

support—emotional, physical, or spiritual—for patients and families during the course of a terminal illness.

In 1975 an international task force established guidelines for hospice programs. Terminally ill people were to be accorded control over the dying process; life-style and personal preference were to be considered in determining treatment goals. Family and friends were to be assisted as well; they, too, suffered emotional, financial, and physical stress. In the process of individualizing treatment for dying patients and their families, hospice workers were also to control patients' physical symptoms. Finally, the staff's reaction to death would also be considered. Providing support for staff members would sustain the quality of their work and help them cope with the stress associated with it.

American hospice programs in the 1990s reflect some of these original ideals, but few programs have been able to implement all of them. Every provider offers assistance to patients and families. Here the similarities end. Care may take place in a special setting or through a traditional health care service. In many cases, programs deviate from original guidelines in that patients' life-styles and preferences are less important than program policies. For example, a patient and family may be reluctant to have death occur at home, but their provider may not offer inpatient services; if the provider does offer such services, admission may be based on medical needs, not patient and family requests. Furthermore, although all hospice programs avow the importance of pain management and symptom control, staff in some programs are inadequately trained to provide these services.

## Accounting for the Popularity of Hospice Care

In the 1960s "the plight of the dying" (Strauss 1975) attracted research and popular interest. Two women, Drs. Cicely Saunders and Elisabeth Kübler-Ross, were among those who asserted that dying had become a social problem, and they recommended an alternative to traditional medical care. Saunders advocated the creation of modern hospices, places that deemphasized medical techniques and employed holistic practices. Kübler-Ross asserted that hospital staff isolated dying patients and made their last days meaningless; she recommended reuniting dying patients with family and friends to give them opportunities to talk about death. The modern hospice envisioned by Saunders appealed to Kübler-Ross as a setting in which she could implement her ideas. Health care professionals were attracted to this new approach to terminal care, and they formed groups—the Yale Study Group being the first of these—to implement hospice programs.

By 1986 hospice programs existed nationwide; three national organizations advocated hospice legislation; and Medicare, Medicaid, and private insurers had established reimbursement structures for hospice services. Yet research indicated that hospice programs showed no resounding benefits for patients or families (Mor 1985); rather, they resembled traditional medical care systems. Politically, the hospice movement had created a supplement, rather than a full-fledged alternative, to traditional medical care.

"Hospice has failed to gain ground. In the past decade, it has developed no national character, no standard criteria for admission into the program, and no generally accepted standard of care" (Sherman and Finn 1987, 20). Hospice workers found that patients referred to hospice programs died before the staff could assist them. As one social worker observed, "You have to be quick and find the ones who aren't quite ready to die and see if they want your assistance in coping with death." Most programs provided support for the dying and their families in their homes and prevented unnecessary hospital admissions. There were exceptions—programs that were able to provide a complete alternative service to hospital care—but they were few and were frequently overlooked by researchers. Nevertheless, these programs maintained the humanitarian emphasis that was central to the movement's original intent.

Many early advocates of hospice care were perplexed by its evolution. How had the enthusiasm to free dying people from unnecessary medical treatments and normalize the dying process resulted in an adjunct to the health care system that seemed little more than a specialized home care service? Three research findings explain the transformation of hospice from a revolutionary way to help dying patients to simply another, albeit specialized, health care service with hospice overtones.

First, and most important, the hospice movement simultaneously reformed and conformed to mainstream medicine. Hospice care humanized (reformed) terminal care, which made it popular with nonphysician health care workers and significant others whose loved ones had died following a protracted illness. It also accommodated (conformed to) policymakers' demands for less costly ways to treat dying patients, which gave it political appeal. Second, the claims of movement leaders that hospice care was a new form of care initiated because the public wanted health care reform were inaccurate. Hospice care was not a new form of care; it had existed in Europe for centuries and in America since the late nineteenth century. Nor was it universally desired by the American public; it was primarily desired by health care workers. Third, dying patients—those with the most to gain—were not involved in the movement. Its mission was determined not by terminally ill patients but by their caregivers; consequently, caregivers seemed more satisfied with hospice services than did dying patients. Research indicated that nurses who worked in hospice programs were less stressed and more satisfied than nurses who worked in traditional health care settings (Vachon 1986). The families of the dying also benefitted from hospice support, particularly when they had access to inpatient services (Greer, Mor, Morris, Sherwood, Kidder, and Birnbaum 1986).

Although the hospice movement has not lived up to its early ideals, it can claim ongoing accomplishments. Its most obvious achievement is that dying patients are less likely to end their days in an intensive care unit surrounded by tubes and machines instead of families and friends. Moreover, the development of hospice programs was timely in regard to the AIDS epidemic and the concomitant social rejection of persons with AIDS (PWAs). Independent hospice facilities for PWAs allow patients who are often rejected by family, friends, and social institutions to receive humane treatment in a comfortable environment during their last days of life. Finally, the hospice movement is international; it has introduced a new method of care for dying patients in Africa, Ireland, West Germany, and many other countries.

## Social Movement Theory

Throughout this book two theoretical themes frame and guide the analysis—social movement and social constructionist theories. Understanding these theories is useful in appreciating what happened to the hospice movement.

Social movements are collective activities intended to bring about social change. The object of change can be a social value, a technology, or both (Back 1989). The study of social movements emphasizes the ideological convictions that inspire participation, the conditions under which movements emerge, and the political processes that facilitate or inhibit movement leaders as they try to achieve their goals. Several theories have dominated research about social movement processes: deprivation theory, stage theory, resource mobilization theory, and new social movement theory. The analysis of the hospice movement incorporates several of these theories, particularly stage theory, resource mobilization, and new social movement theory.

Stage theory offers useful paradigms for describing social movements because it examines the dynamic processes of movements—the way that leaders and participants go about their efforts to influence the larger culture. Stage theory presents "ideal types" and therefore provides a guide rather than a fixed model for explaining social movement processes. Mauss (1975) combined a natural history approach to social problems' rise with a stage theory of social movements' evolution to create a model for examining participants and political processes. According to his model, social movements have life histories of rise and fall much like a bell curve.

A major premise of Mauss's theory is that movements do not arise because of new or increased social problems; rather, a movement emerges as leaders politicize a social condition, and once political goals are achieved the movement declines without having significantly influenced the social condition that caused it. "The cycle begins and ends with individuals and groups on all sides acting out their own interests in response to each other. This is irrespective of objective reality" (Mauss 1975, 59).

Implicit to Mauss's thesis is the assumption that social problems are constructions of reality, not absolute truths. Participants construct problems and the solutions to them in diverse ways based on their differing perspectives. Spector and Kitsuse's (1987) description of claims-making activities, which is in keeping with a social constructionist perspective, is particularly helpful in examining leaders' assertions. Claims-making activities involve the way facts are constructed and presented by reformers. Leaders' claims are not based on objective reality but represent a way to mobilize resources. Leaders' claims are thus analyzed not as facts but as a means of influencing the movement's progress.

Stage theory and claims-making activities are congruent with resource mobilization theory, the dominant theory of social movements for the past two decades. This theory "focuses attention on the ability of the social movement promoters to gain and manipulate resources of power, to organize and recruit members from existing voluntary association networks, and to provide individual incentives or coercion in motivating participation in social movement activities" (Kerbo 1982, 646).

Resource mobilization theorists, too, eschew social conditions, the basis for deprivation theory, as the reason for the emergence of social movements; problematic conditions are constants in society, they argue, and are therefore insufficient to explain the rise of social movements.

Instead resource mobilization theorists take a rational approach to social movement research, examining the movement's organizational structures. According to this method of analysis, a social movement's achievements depend on the way participants organize and acquire resources given the constraints of the political opportunities extant in society (Olson 1965; McCarthy and Zald 1979), and a social movement's organizations, which make up a "social movement industry," are "the glue that holds a social movement together" (Staggenborg 1989, 204).

New social movement theory reintroduces social conditions, participation, and achievements as important components of any attempt to analyze a social movement. Traditionally, deprivation theorists asserted that social strain or frustration explained the emergence and ongoing processes of social movements. As people who were disenfranchised recognized their oppressed condition, it was believed they developed a sense of shared frustration; consequently, groups assembled and developed strategies to ameliorate their circumstances. This point of view characterized the study of the labor movement of the 1930s and 1940s. New social movement theorists believe this rationale fails to explain contemporary movements.

The participants of new social movements, these theorists argue, are individuals who have been adversely affected by modernity (scientific advances, loss of community, loss of meaning in one's work) and/or are members of a new middle class who have rejected capitalistic values (Klandermans and Tarrow 1988). These new middle class participants in social movements are "concerned with cultural issues dealing with questions of individual autonomy and with issues related to new, invisible risks affecting people in more or less similar ways, irrespective of social positions," and they are "social and cultural specialists" (teachers, social workers, artists, economists, lawyers) who oppose technocrats and resist the pressure to conform (Kriesi 1989, 1078).

New social movement theorists support Mauss's thesis that participants' motives are rarely pure. They state that members of a new middle class, employed in nonproductive sectors of society, question the basic economic and political arrangements of industrial society and are predisposed to participate in social movements to advance their own positions. Rohrschneider (1990) found that the participation of the new middle class in the environmental movement, for example, was a way for them to express resentment about their comparatively weak political status.

Resource mobilization theory, according to new social movement theorists, overemphasizes strategy and political process and does not give sufficient credit to the conditions that allow movements to develop or to their ongoing accomplishments. The women's movement, for example, sustains an ongoing mission and its impact persists as feminist organizations continue to alter social attitudes toward women's roles in modern culture.

Finally, contemporary social movements are international, attract a diverse constituency (Kriesi 1989), and are fostered by conditions of affluence rather than crises (Kerbo 1982). The women's movement and ecological movement are examples of new social movements that have become significant internationally. The emergence of these movements does not occur as the result of deprivation, theorists stress, but rather because conditions of affluence allow interest groups to pursue quality-of-life issues.

The hospice movement is consistent with the predictions of new social movement theorists. Its participants were part of a new middle class seeking to improve quality of life. The movement opposed the dehumanizing consequences of modern medical science and supported an anti-authoritarian approach to health care. The hospice movement was also international; Cicely Saunders's model of hospice care has been implemented around the world.

## Social Movement Theory and the Hospice Movement

As noted, social movements are political processes whereby members are recruited, claims are made regarding the need for change, and movement leaders strategize to acquire support from larger bureaucracies. According to Mauss (1975), participants have differing levels of activity and influence on movements, and movements go through stages in which leaders' ability to mobilize resources propels them forward, alters their course, or restricts their progress. There are five possible stages—incipience, coalescence, institutionalization, fragmentation, and demise—and the hospice movement has progressed through all but the last.

**Incipience** During the earliest, or incipient, stage of a social movement, vague, uncoordinated events generate interest in a particular social condition. There is little guidance or control of the movement, no formal organizations; the only groups are formed ad hoc. Informal processes suggest that a serious social problem exists, word spreads regarding this problem, and the movement's rationale is established.

During the incipience of the hospice movement a redefinition of death and dying occurred as certain members of society asserted that the denial of death had become a social problem. The "dying problem" attracted the attention of health care professionals and the lay public, and their activities focused on the way that the individual was denied control of the dying process. "The loss of control experienced by institutionalized, terminally ill patients is a central motif of much thanatological research. Loss of control is seen as loss of dignity. Patients have the right to know their condition, to choose or reject the treatment regimen, to choose or reject attempts to prolong their life, and to decide the disposal of their remains" (Rinaldi and Kearl 1990, 286).

Hospice care was one idea generated by participants in the death with dignity movement, and this movement provided fertile ground for the hospice movement. Saunders and Kübler-Ross became leaders of the death with dignity movement, and ministers and nurses were among its participants. As Saunders's concept of hospice care gained a following, individuals within the death with dignity movement began emphasizing hospice care as means of returning control over death to the dying person.

**Coalescence** A movement coalesces when leaders emerge, groups assemble, and formal organizations are created to do something about the problem. During this phase we observe the way that participants define the problem. The so-called facts about the underlying social problem to be addressed are based on claimants' perceptions of the problem, not objective reality. "Social problems are what people think they are" (Spector and Kitsuse 1987, 73). Or in other words, "That which we perceive to be real becomes real in its effect" (W. I. Thomas, quoted in Landis 1980, 39). Consequently, the claims leaders use to recruit followers and implement reforms need to be examined not as facts but in light of the reality they create and of the way that such claims propel the movement forward.

For example, hospice leaders claimed that hospice care was a response to the public's desire to let death take place at home and to its dissatisfaction with traditional health care. Yet there is little evidence that the public was disgruntled with existing health care services or that they strongly resisted medical treatments. Despite the lack of hard evidence, health care professionals formed planning groups and gained community support to reform what they had redefined as the "unpopular" health care system.

Claiming public demand for reform attracted the attention of the media and policymakers, but it also influenced the way goals were implemented. Because advocates asserted that the public wanted hospices, they did not think that the political forces of mainstream medicine could deter their efforts. Therefore, despite evidence that mainstream medicine co-opted efforts to alter its practices, movement leaders decided to develop hospice programs in hospitals as well as in other health care agencies. This strategy encouraged program development because it allowed hospice care providers to be flexible and to adapt services to different environments, but it also altered services so that programs in hospitals emphasized physical care of dying patients and paid less attention to normalizing the dying process.

**Institutionalization** During the institutional phase a movement experiences its greatest popularity. Laws are enacted, traditional bureaucracies take notice of the movement's cause, and membership is at its greatest. It is also a time when external forces or political opportunities facilitate a co-optation process, as social movement leaders seek larger bureaucracies to assist them in implementing their ideas (Walsh 1978). Once this occurs, the movement moves quickly toward its next stage, fragmentation.

The development of the first few hospice programs attracted the attention of the media and the public, and movement leaders capitalized on it to reinforce their claims that hospice care was an essential and much-desired service. Edward Kennedy and Abraham Ribicoff, U.S. senators seeking ways to expand health care services, were interested in hospice care as a possible new benefit under the Medicare program. Political pressure from hospice supporters forced the National Cancer Institute to support research about hospice care, despite doubts about the efficacy of such services.

Hospice leaders actively sought funding support. Recognizing policymakers' interest in cost-reducing methods of care, they asserted that hospice programs reduced health care costs. Integrating hospice programs with medical environments and appealing to policymakers for funds, however, began to influence the design of hospice services. Bereavement and spiritual support were part of the movement's rhetoric, but most programs had few mechanisms for providing such services. Patients had little control over treatments because hospice workers, trained by route of traditional medical education, had difficulty allowing patient and family control of such decisions. Moreover, programs that were part of traditional health care systems were used to expedite the discharge of difficult patients. The provision of humane care for the dying and their families became a by-product of hospice care rather than its all-consuming goal.

**Fragmentation** The fourth stage in the evolution of a social movement is characterized by fighting among leaders and participants about what has occurred to alter the movement's mission. Participation changes: some members recognize that their goals have been undermined and attempt to reassert their original ideals; those who have benefitted from or approved the compromises attempt to quell the hue and cry; and many participants, particularly those at the periphery of the movement, withdraw, believing that reform efforts have been successful. Social movements are not linear processes with single outcomes; they have multiple outcomes, and different social movement organizations within them achieve dissimilar results.

As policymakers enacted a Medicare hospice benefit and established program standards and reimbursement structures, hospice care providers cried foul. They asserted that policymakers and medical entrepreneurs had colluded to sell out the ideals of the hospice movement. Medicare favored a home care hospice model that made death at home a mandate rather than a patient choice, and reimbursement did not encourage improving bereavement or spiritual services. Older programs failed and new programs were created to meet standards.

Newer leaders in the movement approved the Medicare regulations and asserted that early leaders were unrealistic and had to learn to be more fiscally responsible. As these two groups debated with each other and the government, some hospice advocates begin to withdraw, believing that hospice programs were working—providing a better quality of life for dying patients and their families.

Not all programs were controlled by these political processes. Some providers changed their name from hospice to palliative care unit as a way to reassert their original intent. Others remained to fight, and they set up alternative political organizations to lobby against the funding restrictions placed on hospice programs. Finally, although less financially stable, volunteer community programs persist to this day. These programs were never a part of the movement's political process; the furor regarding limited reimbursement did not interfere with their work and such programs continue to provide nonmedical comfort and support to dying people and their families.

The ongoing achievements of the hospice movement sustain its existence, and therefore it cannot be said that this movement has reached a stage of demise. Several social conditions, such as the increasing number of children who suffer from cancer, sustain collective interest and activities aimed at ameliorating the dying problem.

## Plan of the Book

The intent of this volume is to give the reader an overview of the history of hospice care, of the circumstances that facilitated the popularity of the modern American hospice movement, and of the movement's evolution. Social problems and reformers' solutions to them are rarely unique. Care for the dying and places called hospices have existed since ancient times. The history of care for the dying and the evolution of hospice care in Europe and America are described in chapter 2.

Essential to the emergence of any social movement is an environment that favors collective action. Chapter 3 enables the reader to understand the conditions that fostered the hospice movement's rise in America. These conditions constituted a complex array of societal beliefs, practices, and forces that made possible the emergence of hospice organizations, influenced movement participants' beliefs and strategies, and affected the movement's political processes. The ideas introduced in chapter 3 are transformed into the emergent activities of the 1950s and 1960s discussed in chapter 4.

The way that movement participants go about creating change is at the heart of the analysis of any social movement. Reformers arise to influence and ameliorate social problems, and through their efforts followers gather to support the cause. But it is the use of these humanitarians to serve other purposes (profit motives, efficiency of systems, elevation of the status of a group—that is, self-interest) that gives a social movement its strength and propels it forward. In this process change occurs; some goals are achieved, but many ideals are lost. Chapters 5, 6, and 7 elaborate on the interplay of forces that occurred as movement participants set out to reform care of the dying.

As complex processes, social movements have multiple effects on culture. The broader impact of the hospice movement both in the United States and abroad is explored in chapter 8. Chapter 9 addresses the reasons why the hospice movement has yet to enter the final stage in the evolution of contemporary social movements, demise.

*Chapter 2*

# The Evolution of Hospice Care

Susan was a 48-year-old woman diagnosed as having a malignant tumor of the kidney. Her doctors believed surgery could prolong her life; Susan disagreed. She had witnessed the workings of medical science during the last days of her parents' lives and wanted no part of it for herself; she preferred that nature determine her prognosis. The physician and nurses treating her saw this as a sign of mental illness and requested a psychiatric evaluation. The psychiatrist confirmed her sanity, and the medical team was forced to accept her wish.

Illness was only one of the complicating factors in Susan's case. Divorced and living alone, Susan was a solitary person; her only close relative was a sister who lived thousands of miles away with her own family. Susan did not have a support network to help her with shopping and the other activities of daily life that she could no longer accomplish alone. She wanted to remain in the hospital, but this would have meant a protracted stay, perhaps months, that her insurance would not cover and that she could not afford. A hospice team provided the support network Susan lacked and helped her to remain at home until her death was imminent. She never regretted her choice. Her death was not pleasant—there was pain that the hospice team did its best to alleviate—but it was the way she wanted to complete her life.

The hospice services Susan received are thought by many to be new, but they have roots in the earliest recorded history of health care. The devout and the humanitarian established hospices to mitigate social problems caused by war, pestilence, and poverty. The evolution of hospices through the ages can be said to fall loosely into three time periods: the ancient period, when hospices, along with hospitals, hotels, and hostels, performed many health and social services, including care of the dying; the Middle Ages, when hospices were built as way stations for the crusaders; and the nineteenth century, when hospices were built specifically to care for the terminally ill, owing to the developing emphasis in medical education on scientific treatment and cure. As physicians of became more interested in treatment, they lost interest in the incurable and often discharged them or refused to admit them to the hospital. Consequently, the dying had no place to go. In response, certain religious groups, mostly Christians, built hospices to provide humane care for the terminally ill. With this progression in mind, let us examine the history of hospice from the ancient world to its modern manifestation.

## The Ancient Hospice

It is reasonable to surmise from archaeological finds that the need for separate structures in which to care for the sick or to treat other social problems (such as poverty and homelessness) first developed when humankind formed settled communities (Benoliel 1979). Most such facilities were associated with religious institutions; Egyptians, Orientals, Greeks, and Romans all used their churches or temples as refuges for the sick or for pilgrims. Care of the sick was the responsibility of those believed to have special talents as healers, those who felt it was their religious duty, or diploma physicians who learned their craft based on the scientific knowledge of the time.

Ancient Greek documents indicate the existence of separate structures for plague victims as early as 1134 B.C. (Seplowin and Seravalli 1983). Health care at this time was based on a belief in the powers of Aesculapius, a legendary physician who was deified in the fifth century B.C. Temples for the sick or travel weary were called Aesculapia. Travelers were thought to be under the protection of the god Zeus Xenios, and custom dictated that they be clothed, fed, and entertained with no questions asked until these services were performed. Furthermore, those in need received assistance from primitive healers whose abilities were based on magic, not science.

An early account of a special facility for the dying was recorded in India around 225 B.C. It was opened by the emperor Asoka for religious pilgrims who came to the Ganges River. Their wish was to die there and have their ashes scattered in the river (Davidson 1978). During his reign Asoka built 18 such facilities.

Historically the terms *hospice, hospital, hotel,* or *hostel* were used interchangeably (*hospice* is used as the umbrella term in the following passages here). The etymology of these words derives from the Latin root *hospe,* meaning hospitality (Kohut and Kohut 1984). Care of the dying was usually one of many services offered in ancient hospices, which offered assistance to the sick, the indigent, and the traveler. Although a particular facility might gain a reputation for one or another service, such specialization was idiosyncratic.

Xenodocia—*xenos* meaning guest and *docia* places of reception—for example, were Roman hospices that took in pilgrims, travelers, and all those needing lodging in a strange town (Rosen 1963). Health care as a billable service was also first found in the Roman Empire. Roman military operations fostered the building of these hospices. Public revenues were allocated for their construction, and patients were charged fees.

Christianity (and later Islam) more than other religions saw the care of the sick and dying as a sacred duty. By the end of the fourth century the Church controlled Western medical care (Benoliel 1979). While the healing arts originated in early empires, it was the preaching of Christianity, with its emphasis on love and piety, which led to the growth of hospices for the poor, sick, and homeless (Cohen 1979). "I was sick and ye visited me," was a phrase of Christ's that his followers interpreted as a special responsibility of their belief (Scarborough 1969). Religious healers' motivation to serve the sick was not only to cure their patients; they believed that helping others also saved their own souls. Christian tradition, particularly Catholicism, held preparation for death and the afterlife in high regard; sacrifice in this life earned one rewards in the next.

Church doctrine gave bishops responsibility for providing services for the sick and travel weary. Bishops were instructed to welcome pilgrims into their homes or to find others in the community to perform these services. In A.D. 325 the Council of Nicea, a gathering of religious officials who established Church doctrine, decreed that each bishop should establish a hospice in every city with a cathedral. The emperor Constantine in A.D. 335 supported this dictum by converting Greek Aesculapia to Xenodocia, Christian facilities that received traveling strangers. The Nicean decree was strengthened in A.D. 398 by the Council of Carthage, which urged that these facilities be maintained near churches (Rosen 1963).

Descriptions of Christian hospices built in Greece, Rome, and across Europe are contradictory. Allen (1990) describes an opulent atmosphere, such as is found in the best hotel. Cohen (1979) portrays beautiful exterior structures and courtyards but interior accommodations devoid of comfort and of good ventilation. Stoddard (1978) suggests that guests were carefully attended to but that attendants were ascetics who abstained from creature comforts.

In A.D. 370 Edessa, now al-Ruha, Turkey, Bishop Rabbula created permanent, and apparently quite pleasant, hospice accommodations:

> These were established not simply as hospices for the poor, but also as hospitals for the sick, where they were looked after by a properly organized staff. It would appear that the funding was generous, for according to the bishop's biographer, the food was so good that even those accustomed to being well fed enjoyed the hospital diet, suggesting that not only the poor but also those accustomed to a reasonable standard of living sought the services of xenodocheium. There were two separate establishments, one for men and the other for women, supervised by monks appointed by the bishop. Every effort was made to ensure clean beds and sheets, to attend to the comfort of the patients and to provide the care of an efficient and God-fearing staff of men and women. (Allen 1990, 453)

There are numerous examples of these early hospices. One of the most famous was the Port of Rome begun in A.D. 475 by Fabiola, a Roman matron and a disciple of Jerome during the time of Emperor Julian the Apostate. Fabiola "witnessed the monasteries in the Holy Land, and brought this concept back with her to Italy, not only supporting hospices financially, but also serving as a nurse herself" (Kastenbaum 1991, 108). The shelters she built were open to travelers as well as the sick or dying (Corr and Corr 1983).

In Ireland (A.D. 500) Saint Bridget provided care for the lame, lost, sick, and dying, and Garrison's (1929) medical history tells of the mountain Xenodocia at Mount Cenis (A.D. 825) and the Great Saint Bernard (A.D. 962), located in the Swiss Alps and staffed by Augustine monks. The latter facility, which still exists, was the famous snow-topped refuge where Saint Bernard dogs were credited with saving the lives of travelers who became lost or sick while journeying through the mountain pass. Thomas Aquinas reports of seeking shelter in such hospices during his travels. Garrison goes on to report that, "it became the ambition of many a prince or landgrave to found a Xenodocium pauperium debilium et infirmium" (119–20)—a hospice for the sick and infirmed.

Moslems also saw care for the sick as a religious duty, and they built hospices throughout the Islamic world. Their knowledge of medical care was obtained from the ancient Greeks. Moreover, they are credited with sustaining classic Greek medical knowledge, adding to it, and being the conduit for reintroducing its scientific principles to Western culture during the Renaissance.

Unlike the health care based on religious beliefs of medieval Christian culture, the Moslems created facilities that emphasized scientific principles. "In Baghdad, Cairo, Damascus, Cordova, and many other cities under their control, they provided ample, and frequently luxurious, accommodations" (Cohen 1979, 16). By A.D. 1160 a visitor to Baghdad reported finding no less than 60 infirmaries. Islam's high standards for health care persisted until the fifteenth century.

## The Crusades and the Rise of Hospices

The Crusades, which began late in the eleventh century and continued for several hundred years, are a milestone in hospice history. Institutions called hospices became popular during the Crusades, and it is these ancient facilities with which people are most familiar. There were 750 hospices in England by the thirteenth century, 40 in Paris, and 30 in Florence (McNulty and Holderby 1983). Hospices were way stations for weary travelers and well known to crusaders.

The hospices of the Middle Ages often featured expensive tapestries and stained glass windows. Every effort was made to create an attractive appearance by including courtyards with gardens in their design (DuBois 1980). Yet in keeping with Catholic belief, which then encouraged personal sacrifice, the wards were bare, with only the simplest of beds to accommodate patients or travelers. Ventilation was also poor, owing to the stained glass windows (Cohen 1979).

Crusading knights helped the religious to build hospices. The Hospitaller Knights established hospices in Europe and Syria, and the Order of Saint John in Jerusalem created the well-known structures in Rhodes and Malta as well as other hospices in their command scattered throughout Europe (Cohen 1979). These hospices were not only for male crusaders; the Saint Mary Magdalene Hospice was devoted to the care of women (Kutscher 1983).

The weary crusader struggling to return to home found comfort and shelter in the welcoming, peaceful hospices scattered across Europe and the Holy Lands.

On doorways are the elaborately decorated shields of the various national orders of the Hospitaller Knights of Saint John; beyond iron palings are inner courts filled with blooming oleanders, oranges, and geraniums. In the great hall "Our Lords the Sick" were received. They were gently washed and carried to beds, each with its own curtain around it, and there they were served by the noble knights themselves. All personnel here, the traveler reads, were under oath of personal poverty, and even the acceptance of gifts from grateful patients was forbidden. The knights and attendants ate in their own quarters, far plainer fare; and if they were unkind to patients or if they neglected their needs in any way, they were put on bread and water for a week and whipped. (Stoddard 1978, 26–28)

## The Rise of Medicine

The health care at hospices from ancient times through the Crusades was usually provided by religious caregivers. Although they were willing helpers, their treatment methods did little to reduce the incidence of disease. Church-led medical practice was ruled by superstition, and clergy, who were the diploma physicians, held back scientific progress particularly during the latter half of the Middle Ages. Church dogma regarding medical treatments was rooted in the belief in saving souls and doing good works, not in an understanding of physiology. One way religious beliefs interfered with medical practice is evidenced by an edict of 1163, which forbade any surgery that caused blood to be shed. The body was the sacred repository of the soul, and any surgery was a desecration (Bronowski 1973).

The Reformation resulted in the transfer of medical authority to secular institutions, and health care became the domain of scientists. Out of the eighteenth century, in contrast to the Church-dominated control of intellectual growth during medieval times, came the encouragement of intellectual liberalism. "Enlightened monarchs, like Josef II of Austria, Catherine II of Russia, and Frederick the Great of Prussia encouraged new concepts, experimental study and discovery, giving an enormous impetus to scientific culture" (Castiglione 1947, 578). While many diseases remained incurable, attempts were made to construct systemic theories that explained important physiological and pathological phenomena.

The expansion of scientific knowledge and the emphasis on research and cure influenced the purpose of hospitals. As scientific inquiry progressed, specialization occurred in facilities that had been multifunctional. For example, separate institutions were created to treat different types of illness, such as mental illness or small pox.

During the seventeenth century the creation of new hospices was rare; older hospices were renamed hospitals and others ceased to exist. There were, however, a few exceptions to this trend. Saint Vincent De Paul opened hospices in Paris for the care of orphans and the poor, sick, and dying, and he organized the Sisters of Charity to staff them. Baron Von Stein of Prussia witnessed the work of Saint Vincent and encouraged a Protestant pastor in his hometown to found Kaiserworth Hospice, which was run by an order of Protestant sisters. Both orders sent representatives to the Crimea during the 1850s, where they worked with Florence Nightingale.

As secular influences began to dominate medical thinking, university-trained physicians sought to improve their status and hospitals became their laboratory. Before the 1800s medicine was a natural art performed by apothecaries, midwives, barber surgeons, and diploma physicians (Freidson 1970a). Diploma physicians were not viewed as experts or accorded high status; midwives, apothecaries, and lay healers were their equals, and the public received health care from their preferred healer in their own home. Those who sought medical care in hospitals were often poor and unable to afford other services.

As knowledge of human physiology increased, university-trained physicians applied a scientific approach to treating disease and sought to establish their credibility with the public. Research-minded physicians working in hospitals believed that their function was to cure diseases, not to provide supportive services for the dying poor or respite for weary travelers. Despite physicians' efforts to change the purpose and function of hospitals, however, they remained places where infection and death were the more common outcome. The poor were forced to accept these services, and the general public did not value the care offered there.

Industrialization played a part in the expansion of European hospitals and the demand for physicians. Migrants from the countryside who came to work in city factories soon fell victim to epidemics such as typhoid fever, tuberculosis, and other diseases associated with overcrowded and unsanitary living conditions. Without family supports they ended up in hospitals, which expanded to accommodate the increased demand. The new diploma physician saw the hospital as a place to perform clinical studies and autopsies (Bullough and Bullough 1972).

To improve their image, physicians began to control access to hospitals. They discouraged hospital use by patients with chronic, incurable, or terminal conditions; individuals seeking shelter or comfort during their last hours were refused admission. Physicians not only perceived care of the dying as being outside the scope of medical work, they viewed death as a threat to their professional advancement. The university-trained physician did not want his reputation tarnished by failures. As early as 1808 attention was drawn to the fact that certain medical practitioners referred to the Dundee Royal Infirmary patients who were far advanced in illness with no prospect of recovery. A medical officer in one hospital wrote, "What opinion would the public form of the skill of medical attendants in the house, if upon looking at the annual reports it should appear that the cases of death were to those of recovery as three to one" (Rosen 1963, 29).

Almshouses and workhouses were created to house the chronically ill, poor, or dying who were unwelcome in hospitals. Although these institutions represented an attempt to serve a public need, they were rarely comfortable or pleasant. Almshouses and workhouses were overcrowded and primitive attempts to control the poor while appearing to offer them services. Moreover, because the number of such facilities was limited, individuals were as likely to end up in the streets, and perhaps they preferred that fate. Charles Dickens depicted workhouses as terrible places. A character in *Our Mutual Friend* states her preference for death in the fields over admission to a workhouse.

The changes in medical practice that began in the eighteenth and nineteenth centuries were compounded in the early part of the twentieth century by the development of such technologies as the X ray and radiation. A biomedical model of disease developed that applied reductionist principles to the care of the sick and the study of illness (Benoliel 1979). From this perspective, disease was defined as a deviation from certain physical and biochemical norms. The objectification of the doctor/patient relationship, with its emphasis on diagnosis and cure, further distanced the physician and his laboratory (the hospital) from human problems. Medicine developed specialty practices, but thanatology was not one of them, and until the 1950s few if any efforts were made to educate physicians about death and dying.

## The Revival of Hospice Care in Europe

During the nineteenth century hospices experienced a rebirth as they began to specialize in the care of terminally ill people. There were two reasons for their resurgence. First, the horrors of the potato famine in Ireland (and of poverty in other countries) gave rise to a need for special care. Second, the clergy became aware that secular hospitals tended to send incurables to other institutions that were even less sympathetic to their physical needs than were hospitals (Corr and Corr 1983).

Our Lady's Hospice, which opened in 1879, was the first facility created under religious auspices to provide palliative care for dying people. Reports on the development of Our Lady's Hospice conflict, but it appears from the majority of documents (Stoddard 1978; McNulty and Holderby 1983; Kohut and Kohut 1984; Corr and Corr 1983; and Fulton and Owen 1981) that it was inspired by Sister Mary Aikenhead, a member of the Irish Sisters of Charity. Sister Mary had worked with Florence Nightingale and was familiar with the Saint Vincent De Paul hospices in France. She considered death to be life's final pilgrimage, and she used the term *hospice*, associated with the pilgrims of yore, for her new facility (Kohut and Kohut 1984).

Although Sister Mary conceived the notion of a hospice for the terminally ill, she never lived to see her idea implemented; the opening of Our Lady's in Harold Cross, Dublin, took place 21 years after her death. The choice of setting was apt, as the following quote from an 1835 issue of the *Dublin Penny Journal* shows: "A pleasant village . . . the air in this neighborhood has long been considered particularly favorable to invalids; and the village has therefore been much frequented by persons in a delicate state of health" (quoted in McNulty and Holderby 1983, 9–10).

The spread of Sister Mary's philosophy led to the creation of hospices in England, France, Australia, and the United States. In 1874 a Madame Garnier organized the Women of Calvary to found houses to care for the dying destitute in Paris and in others parts of France (Koff 1980). The far-reaching spread of hospice programs resulted in the building of the Sacred Hearts Hospice in Australia. This facility was opened in 1890 by a branch of the Sisters of Charity (McNulty and Holderby 1983).

In England hospice facilities flourished toward the beginning of the twentieth century. Many of these early hospices survive to this day and were part of the modern British hospice movement. In 1891 William Hoare of the Merchant Bankers of London appealed for money to establish a home for the terminally ill. This facility, the Hostel of God, run by the Anglican sisters, still exists independent of the National Health Service. Saint Luke's House of the Dying Poor in Bayswater, London, which was managed by the Methodist committee, opened in 1893; it was here that Cicely Saunders, a founder of the modern hospice movement, volunteered in 1948 while waiting admission to medical school. This facility's founder, unlike most hospices of the era, was a physician, Howard Bassett, who sought to treat each of his patients as a "human microcosm, with its own characteristics, its own life history, intensely interesting to itself and some small surrounding circle" (DuBoulay 1984, 61). The following description of Saint Luke's House for the Dying Poor appeared in an English review entitled "Havens of Peace": "The primary object of the institution is the reception and care without payment of persons, who prior to admission thereto, are stated by the medical officer of the institution to be suffering from any disease or injury from which, in his belief, the death of such a person is to be apprehended in no distant date" (Downie 1973, 1069).

Elizabeth Fry, a member of English Sisters of Charity, fought for hospital and prison reform, and she developed hospices through her religious group in London. One of these hospices, Saint Joseph's in London, opened at the turn of century, and it was at this hospice that Saunders took her first position as medical officer in 1958.

## The Rise of Medical Care in the United States

In America, physician domination and specialization of hospitals as places to treat those deemed curable paralleled the European experience, except that it occurred 50 years later (Starr 1982). The case was the same regarding the sorry state of services for the indigent poor. In 1736 the New York Public Workhouse was reported to have allocated one of its rooms to the care of the sick (MacEachern 1957), and in many towns almshouses were the only form of medical facility available. The overcrowding and squalor of such places did little to improve the health of those forced to seek shelter there. Hospices were created at the end of the nineteenth century to assist dying cancer patients who were unwelcome or poorly treated in hospitals and workhouses.

Originally medical care in America was the clergy's responsibility, but this soon changed as barber surgeons, midwives, and diploma physicians replaced them. As was the case in Europe, university-trained physicians were in the minority among healers of the seventeenth and eighteenth centuries. In 1775 the United States had a total of some 3,500 "physicians," but only 400 held university medical degrees (Ackernecht 1968).

Educational standards for American university-trained physicians declined following the Civil War. Their popularity also diminished, and the public's preference for natural healers increased. In contrast, European university-trained physicians were gaining status. U.S. medical educators decided that they needed to improve their image. Members of the Council on Medical Education and Hospitals, established in 1905, began a rigorous study of the existing 160 medical schools. Attempts at reform, however, were only half hearted until the publication in 1911 of the Flexner report, a widely publicized document that identified the inadequacies of the majority of medical schools. This report spurred the improvement of educational standards for physicians, and many medical schools were forced to close. By 1955 only 75 accredited schools remained (MacEachern 1957).

The massive reforms in training instituted in the United States led to a physician domination of the U.S. health care system not paralleled in Europe. Both Freidson (1970a) and Starr (1982) have described the success of the solo practice, fee-for-service physician in dominating health care services. Physicians' ability to control access to medical care altered the purpose of hospitals. The transformation of medical education went hand in hand with improvements in American hospital conditions, so that doctors (and nurses) came to the hospital for their training. American medicine, once it became hospital centered, did so to a greater degree than in other countries. The growth of insurance coverage in the United States during the 1930s further encouraged hospital use (Bullough and Bullough 1972).

## The Development of American Hospices

The origin of American hospices is rarely acknowledged in modern hospice literature. One early chronicler of the modern hospice movement, for example, described the development of hospices for the terminally ill in Ireland and their spread to other continents; he concludes by saying hospices continued to develop in the early part of this century, "but without any impact on the United States until the 1960s" (Rossman 1977, 83).

There are several reasons for this oversight. First, America had fewer hospices than Europe, and those that existed were viewed negatively by the public. "Death house," was a common euphemism for such places. Second, the leaders of the hospice movement perceived the older facilities as places where treatment ceased; they saw modern hospice care as a vehicle for a new treatment method. Finally, religious caregivers who ran the existing hospices did not actively pursue integration with the new reformers; for the most part they were uninterested in the movement's political goals, such as gaining access to insurance reimbursement or integrating with mainstream medicine.

The first American hospices, like their European counterparts, were created because modern hospitals were unable or unwilling to provide services for terminally ill patients. Unlike in Europe, terminal care facilities in America specialized in the care of dying cancer patients. The first American hospices appeared around the turn of the century and followed the religious tradition of caring for the dying when medicine chose to relinquish control. As in Europe, religious orders were founded to look after dying persons and their families.

Rose Hawthorne Lathrop, Nathaniel Hawthorne's daughter, was a prominent advocate of hospice care for cancer patients during the late 1890s. As with many other individuals who became interested in the care of dying people, Rose Hawthorne Lathrop personally experienced a loss with the death of her child. This made her sensitive to the needs of the dying and their survivors, and she organized a group of women called the Servants of Relief of Incurable Cancer. Although she started her work as a lay person, when her husband died she decided to take religious vows. Her title became Mother Alphonsa, and her organization became the Dominican Sisters of Hawthorne (Guenette 1989).

At first Mother Alphonsa and her sisters provided home care services. As her work became known and appreciated, she received donations to build an inpatient facility. Mother Alphonsa chose to imitate European hospices for terminally ill patients, and she built Saint Rose's Hospice in lower Manhattan. The Dominican Sisters of Hawthorne created six other hospice facilities in various cities, including New York, Denver, Philadelphia, and Saint Paul. Several of these facilities still exist, continuing to care for terminally ill cancer patients.

The services provided by these first American hospices had much in common with the modern hospice programs begun in the early 1970s. Separated by nearly a century, both groups of providers observed the inadequate care terminally ill cancer patients received in traditional medical environments and created an alternative method of care.

The two groups differed, however, in their philosophies on family involvement. Modern hospice programs were designed to include the family in the dying process. In contrast, places like Saint Rose's admitted patients from hospitals or homes and then limited family visits to a few times each week. Early providers believed that the family had suffered enough and should be given permission to relinquish the task of caregiving to the sisters who saw it as their duty. Among the original hospice facilities still functioning visitation restrictions have been eased, but the underlying philosophy persists.

Although they have no particular organization to unite them, hospices such as Saint Rose's perpetuate the Christian religious tradition of caring for the sick and dying, and their services are still free. These hospices never sought insurance reimbursement; instead, they have relied on donations. In keeping with their mission to alleviate family stress, they refuse financial gifts from the immediate members of patients' families.

Until the 1970s, when intermediate care facilities were forced to accept the New York State Board of Health's regulations, hospices in New York discouraged medical intervention. Once a patient came to them, few efforts were made to diagnose or treat new physical symptoms. Patients were not forbidden treatment, but neither were they encouraged to request medical services. As the definition of what constituted medical care expanded (treatment for alcoholism, infertility, and the symptoms of aging), terminal care was incorporated into the health care industry and providers had to conform to the mandates of state and national regulatory boards. As part of the "medical industrial complex" hospices had to hire professional staff, such as medical directors and social workers, to oversee patient care. Despite regulatory changes, patients at these hospices who seek extensive medical intervention must obtain it outside the facility.

Lack of technology has never affected the popularity of these hospices with patients and families, and those residing at these facilities do not appear to have any greater degree of discomfort than do those who receive traditional medical care (Siebold 1987). The atmosphere is peaceful and reminds one of Stoddard's (1978) description of the tranquility of the mountain hospices built during the Crusades. Unlike those ancient way stations whose doors were open to all in need, admission to these hospices can take months. Because they are oversubscribed, they require medical proof (usually in the form of X ray and tumor reports) attesting that the patient has a life expectancy of less than six months. Once a patient is accepted, however, there is no limit on the amount of time he or she can stay.

One well-known example of a facility that combines hospice-like care with traditional medical treatment is Calvary Hospital, opened in New York City in 1899. Calvary, like Saint Rose's or Rosary Hill, emphasizes palliative care and spiritual comfort during the last days of life, but it also has the capacity to perform medical techniques that will reduce physical discomfort or provide patient and family peace of mind in knowing that medical science's capacity for cure has been explored. Although now categorized as a specialty hospital, its origins resemble those of hospices.

Calvary Hospital was founded by Catherine McPardan. She began her work by bringing together a group of Irish Catholic laywomen and providing in-home support for the dying poor in lower Manhattan. Eventually, they were able to build a hospital on Featherbed Lane in the Bronx. As the neighborhood changed and the demand for Calvary's services increased, a new facility was built, also in the Bronx. For many years it was staffed by several orders of Catholic nuns, including the Dominican Sisters of the Sick Poor, the Dominicans of Bleauvelt, and the Little Company of Mary.

During its early history Calvary was a free hospital, but this changed during the 1960s when the Medicare and Medicaid programs created reimbursement structures for chronic care. (A similar example is the Dominican Sisters of the Sick Poor, who had provided free home care services. When Medicare began reimbursing for home care services this order became a visiting nurse service eligible for Medicare. It did, however, continue to offer in-home support free for patients who were ineligible for Medicare or unable to pay for services.) Although charging for services made Calvary Hospital a business rather than a religious mission, the emphasis of care was still comfort, not cure, with only minimal use of modern medical technology.

Today Calvary operates as it did at the turn of the century, as a cancer hospital with a hospice philosophy. Patients are admitted only when they are terminally ill; a physician's prognosis, or educated guess, is required. The majority of patients remain at Calvary until death, but there are times when patients outlive their prognosis and are discharged home. Since the 1980s Calvary has developed home care services to facilitate patients' transition from hospital to home.

The atmosphere at Calvary appears at first to be reminiscent of a typical community hospital. A closer look reveals important differences. Each patient has a private room. The facility is spotless, and space is allocated in such a way that the signs and smells of sickness are not concentrated or overwhelming to the visitor. Staff members visit patients frequently, not to assess the improvement or deterioration of their condition but to offer support. Although treatments are not encouraged, neither are they discouraged. As one Calvary physician states, "Over the years we have tried not to deny patients access to any kind of care that they think appropriate" (Cimino 1983, 227). The emphasis is on comfort and spiritual peace for patient and family, but if someone strongly desires treatment up to the last day of life, Calvary will try to provide it.

Employees at Calvary were involved in the modern hospice movement during its early years. It is one of the facilities where health care workers were encouraged to assemble and learn about the ideas of Cicely Saunders and Elisabeth Kübler-Ross. Nonetheless, Calvary neither participated in the movement's political process nor attempted to transform itself into a modern hospice. It continues to be licensed as a specialty hospital and a long-term care facility.

## The New Hospice Movement

Facilities such as Calvary Hospital and Saint Rose's Hospice continue to provide institutional care for the terminally ill. Few such facilities were created in America, and by the 1930s it became common practice for dying patients to end their days in hospitals or nursing homes. The modern hospice movement did not emerge from within these older programs. It was terminal care practices in hospitals and nursing homes that attracted the concern of scholars and nonphysician health care workers during the 1950s and 1960s. They believed that hospitals and nursing homes were ill-prepared to care for dying patients and, worse yet, mistreated them. Terminally ill patients were "transferred back and forth between hospital and nursing home because 'this patient doesn't belong here' " (Wass 1979, 163).

The modern hospice movement saw itself as new and unique, yet the social problem it sought to address—mistreatment of the dying—was the same one identified by nineteenth-century reformers like Rose Hawthorne Lathrop. Participants in the modern hospice movement differed from early providers of hospice care in seeking to reform traditional medical practice.

When Saunders and Kübler-Ross first began to speak out against health care practices that dehumanized or ignored the dying person, the sisters at Calvary and other facilities came to listen. These religious devotees helped spread the word about new ways to ease the physical, spiritual, and psychological pain of the dying, but that was the extent of their involvement. Facilities such as Calvary and Saint Rose's, philosophically rooted in the religious beliefs of their founders, were uninterested in the political struggles of the hospice movement. Hospice movement leaders saw these older institutions as representing the end of treatment; they wanted to reform medical care and add new treatments. This fundamental difference between the missions of the older, established hospices and new the movement for reform is largely responsible for the tendency of the latter to ignore the existence of the former.

# Chapter 3

# Social Conditions That Fostered the Hospice Movement

The hospice movement has been depicted as a grass roots reform movement, a response to rising consumer demand for more control over health services; a religious movement, an attempt to return spirituality to the dying process; and a professional movement, an effort by nonphysician health care workers to rebel against authoritarian hospital systems. Each characterization is accurate because the hospice movement is not a single-issue movement that arose from a discrete set of circumstances. It has incorporated different perspectives, was triggered by a number of conditions, and attracted participants by virtue of one or all of these conditions.

The social conditions that supported the hospice movement's rise in the 1960s and influenced its course in the 1970s can be divided into four categories: the growing popular interest in death, the increasing attention to quality of life, the expanding capacities of medical science, and the escalating cost of health care. This chapter provides an overview of these conditions and the ways they affected the hospice movement. The first two categories fostered the development of the hospice movement; the last two simultaneously supported and altered the movement's goals.

## Social Conditions: An Overview

The hospice movement developed in an environment that favored collective action. According to Mauss (1975), the liberal atmosphere that existed during the 1960s resulted in more social movements than any other time in history, including the civil rights movement, the women's movement, and the gay rights movement. The hospice movement was among these collective activities, and its cause, to ameliorate the plight of the dying, was consistent with increased efforts to improve conditions for all members of society.

More specifically, the hospice movement emerged during a time when death was at the forefront of American attention. John F. Kennedy's assassination in 1963 created public and scientific interest in death, dying, and grief. Prior to Kennedy's death, these topics received little popular attention; his assassination brought them to the fore as Americans witnessed on television Kennedy's last moments in Dallas and his funeral in Washington. The Vietnam War, known as the living room war for being the first to enter people's homes daily on television, also brought death to the public's attention.

Popular interest in death, dying, and grief was a necessary condition for the emergence of the hospice movement. Social surveys of the public's attitudes and behaviors toward death became common. As research about death proliferated, a new field of study, thanatology, was created (*thanatos* is the Greek word for death).

The desire for meaningful work and the demand for specialized services that intensified in the 1960s also supported the development of the hospice movement. Hospice philosophy averred that workers' needs were as important as their clients' needs and that dying patients and their families required a special form of service, tailored to the particular stresses that each faced during a terminal illness.

The expansion of medical technology was the most complex influence on the hospice movement, because it both encouraged and inhibited the development of hospice programs. The advanced ability of medical science to sustain life raised ethical issues among health care professionals about the morality of keeping people alive when there was no hope of cure, and this encouraged a search for humane solutions. At the same time, some feared that ceasing treatment might encourage some form of genocide, and they opposed efforts to control access to medical treatments. Hospice leaders attempted to strike a balance and appeal to both sides of this argument.

Finally, the cost of health care during the latter half of the twentieth century rose at such an alarming rate that policymakers sought ways to reduce expenditures. This last factor, although not central to the ideology or emergence of the hospice movement, had the greatest impact on the hospice industry. Hospice providers' willingness to be cost-effective made them attractive to policymakers seeking less expensive treatments and to medical entrepreneurs seeking profitable ways to expand the health care industry.

## The Denial of Death

During the 1950s and 1960s a body of knowledge developed asserting that the denial of death had become a common social phenomenon in Western culture. Advocates of this viewpoint cited funerary rituals, attitudes toward disease, religious beliefs, and the way people spoke about death as evidence of this new attitude of denial. The belief that this denial was a social problem stirred some people to a cause, "the plight of the dying" (Strauss 1975). One way to combat this death denial was hospice care, through which dying patients and their families would be encouraged to acknowledge death and would receive support to cope with its effects.

**An Unacceptable Event in the Life Cycle**   Semantic practices were one source of evidence used to support assertions that Western culture denied death. Euphemisms for "died" or "deceased," such as "passed on," or "at rest," were construed as ways to avoid talking about, and thus avoid accepting, death. At one Boston hospital the staff referred to a patient's death by saying he or she had been "transferred to Allen Street" (Mor, Greer, and Kastenbaum 1988). The use of embalming fluid, putty, cotton, and cosmetics to make the dead appear more life-like served as further proof that Americans wanted to avoid the reality of death (Cohen 1979).

Research on changed behavior toward the dying and negative attitudes toward illness were other sources of evidence for those claiming that Western culture was death denying. Phillipe Ariès's (1974) research of funeral practices concluded that a slow shift had occurred in Western attitudes and behaviors toward death and that American culture played an important part in this change. According to Ariès, before the twelfth century there existed "tamed death." Death had meaning only for the one who was dying; it was usually swift, or there might be a brief period to reflect and organize one's affairs. Under these circumstances death was a customary fact of human destiny, and the average person neither feared nor avoided the dying process. From the twelfth to the eighteenth centuries practices and attitudes changed as the time to prepare for death extended. Family and friends were included in the dying process, and practices such as death-bed vigils became more common.

Cemeteries and death rituals were considered neither strange nor frightening but rather central to daily life. It was common practice for villagers to spend time in burial grounds, dancing or engaging in other social activities. In fact, cemeteries were often located in the center of town so exposure to them was unavoidable. The lack of concern about separating the living from corpses, according to Ariès, posed serious health threats. Primitive water systems, unprotected from the contaminating effects of nearby cemeteries, spread disease.

During the eighteenth century death became a romantic preoccupation. The starving artist, dying of consumption in his garret, spitting blood into a delicate lace handkerchief, exemplified the romanticization of death. This macabre interest in dying and death increased the importance of funeral rituals for survivors. Mourning practices, particularly for widows, came into being. It was common practice for family and friends of the dying to keep their knowledge of the person's impending death from him or her. The dying were consequently unlikely to be involved in the social rituals preceding death.

It was not until the twentieth century that our current social dilemma emerged. Death became an unacceptable, shameful event that transpired in a sterile atmosphere. Physicians preferred to treat their patients in institutions, and people were more likely to die in a hospital bed, isolated from families and friends. Death-bed vigils became antiquated, and family participation was discouraged as dying people were ministered to by technical experts.

Ariès concluded that as a result of these practices, a death-denying culture emerged. As knowledge about medical science advanced, the time of death could be more accurately predicted, and people avoided observing the dying process or participating in death rituals. Allowing technicians the role of overseers of death reinforced the practice of not telling patients about their impending demise. Segregating dying patients from the living and obscuring death's occurrence by sustaining life through artificial means distanced people from the reality of death. "Death has been dissected, cut to bits by a series of little steps, which finally make it impossible to know which step was the real death" (Ariès 1974, 88).

The changed attitudes described by Ariès did not include an examination of cultural attitudes toward disease, but here, too, shame and secrecy were said to surround processes not within human control. As death commonly comes at the end of these illnesses, the shame attached to the disease might influence attitudes and behaviors toward death itself.

Historical evidence suggests that as far back as the medieval period disease was viewed as a punishment for sins (Castiglione 1947). When the plagues ravaged Europe the sick were often treated with revulsion and judged as somehow deserving their fate (Seplowin and Seravalli 1983). It was believed that the sufferer's moral failings contributed to his or her plight. Thus, the sick person dealt not only with despair over illness but also suffered feelings of shame for having contracted a disease.

Today cancer is sometimes believed to be caused by individual failings. One patient blamed herself for having acquired her disease because she did not verbalize her feelings. The feelings, according to this woman, resulted in stomach ulcers, which then became cancer. AIDS patients are also often blamed for their illness. Promiscuous sexual practice or drug addiction, contributing factors in the spread of AIDS, are presented as if they caused the disease.

Increased secularization, according to some scholars, is what led to death-denying practices. An earlier, church-dominated society conceived of life as a time of sacrifice to earn a heavenly reward. The absence of strong spiritual ties in the modern world diminished the importance of preparing oneself to meet one's maker and, therefore, the importance of death. "We live in a society that increasingly finds itself without a creedal or mythic framework in which to understand life and interpret death" (Wass 1979, 40). Hinton (1977) found that in England 25 percent of the population disclaimed any religious belief, while 50 percent did not believe in an afterlife. His results were consistent with American religious beliefs in the 1970s.

Examination of contemporary funeral practices supported the idea that as a culture we did not value death or the dying process. Evelyn Waugh's satiric depiction of funeral practices in *The Loved One* (1948) portrayed funerals as commercialized and dehumanized events. Over time these fictional allegations were supported by research about the mortuary industry. Jessica Mitford's *The American Way of Death* (1963) assessed funeral methods and their costs, and she suggested that morticians, not the bereaved, benefitted from such practices.

**Institutional Causes of Death Denial**  Another interpretation of the problem was suggested by Fox (1979), who stated that sociological evidence does not support the idea that Western culture is death denying. Fox argued that it is the environment in which death occurs (hospitals and nursing homes) that gives the appearance of denial.[1] Blauner (1966) stated that relegating the dying to special institutions reduced their disruptive effect on the ongoing business of society. Studies of medical environments support Fox's contention that these environments isolate the dying person and dehumanize the process and that staff, patient, and family are influenced by systemic forces (Fox 1979; Glaser and Strauss 1965; Kübler-Ross 1969; and Sudnow 1967). Freidson (1970b) explains this point of view: "A significant amount of behavior is situational in nature . . . that people are constantly responding to the organized pressures of the situation they are in at any particular time, that what they are is not completely but more their present than their past, and what they do is more an outcome of the pressures of the situation they are in than of what they have earlier internalized" (90).

Medical environments, with their emphasis on preserving life, encourage staff members to avoid and deny the reality of death. Furthermore, encouraging staff to discuss death might impede their ability to maintain an emphasis on life supports. Families for the most part take their cues from medical staff and do not contest the emphasis on treatments. As death in hospitals became more common, families became unfamiliar with and therefore reluctant to observe the dying process.

Glaser and Strauss (1965) studied the behavior of medical staff toward dying patients, and they found that patients who died in the hospital were abandoned by staff and left to struggle with complex feelings about their condition without much support. Staff communication and interaction with patients diminished as the inevitability of their death became obvious. The nearer to death a patient was, the less often their physicians visited and the slower ancillary staff were to answer call bells.

More extreme, even ghoulish, is the behavior documented in Sudnow's study (1967) of staff response to the death of a patient.

Despite the fact that it is routinely done, body wrapping is regarded by aides and orderlies throughout the hospital as an unpleasant task, and while these personnel come to do it with no special fear, they do not characteristically look forward to it. In fact, they systematically attempt to avoid the task. One common devise at county is to pretend that the patient has not died, and if necessary and possible, try to camouflage his death by making him look alive. If they succeed, aides or orderlies can manage to pass off the body for the next shift, which, when rounds are made, will discover it and be responsible for wrapping it. The body is camouflaged by propping the head up,

closing the eyes to feign the appearance of sleep, keeping intravenous solutions flowing, and screening off the body so that bypassing personnel, e.g.,
nurses, doctors, will not notice the dead body. (82)

Leaders of the hospice movement knew about studies regarding the
negative effect of medical environments. In the early stages of the movement they used data about the inability of hospital staff to care for the
terminally ill to support their call for hospice programs, and some warned
that these programs should be separate from hospitals. As the movement
progressed, however, this warning was heard less frequently. Instead
providers insisted that hospice care could take place in various settings.

**Death and Grief: A Psychological Perspective** Research on the
psychological impact of death and the stress of not being able to talk
openly about also supported claims that death denial the denial of death
was a social problem. Clinicians stated that the fears of dying people
needed to be addressed and that the grief of their family and friends could
lead to psychological and physical difficulties. A longitudinal study of
widowers' emotional and physical responses to loss conducted from 1957
to 1966, for instance, found that widowers were more likely than their
married male counterparts to suffer from physical disease, and sometimes
death, in the first year following their spouse's death (Parkes, Benjamin,
and Fitzgerald 1969).

During the 1960s and 1970s, clinical studies increased. These studies
examined dying and grief both as a natural, but emotionally stressful,
experience and as a pathological process requiring treatment. Clinicians
such as Kastenbaum (1991), Kübler-Ross (1969), Maddison and Walker
(1967), and Silverman (1986) studied the individual's reaction to death
and recommended professional and self-help techniques. Their recommendations will be further explored when we examine the emergence of
the death with dignity movement in chapter 4.

**Countertrends: Is Death Denied?** As death and dying became an
"in" topic, some social scientists suggested that claims that we had
become a death-denying culture were exaggerated. "The assertion that
death is a taboo topic in America has been repeated so often by so many
people, in so many contexts, that one begins to believe it must surely,
somewhere, be engraved in stone—the revealed word of the gods"
(Lofland 1975, 10). Nettler (1967) is more critical, suggesting that

research on the subject of death has little to offer: "The psychoanalytic and literary death-metaphors, so conveniently adopted by some sociologists, will receive any data as confirmation and none as their negation. The reader is entertained. There has been a verbal massage and one feels better, or worse, although he remains ignorant" (337).

Participants in the hospice movement were not unaware of such critiques, in fact they often agreed with them. A common phrase adopted by supporters of hospice care was "hospice is about living, not dying," thus suggesting that they had no morbid fascination with death and were not simply an offshoot of the faddist interest in death and dying.

## Quality of Life:
## An Emerging Concept

During the latter half of the twentieth century a new phrase, "quality of life," became popular. It referred to improving one's life-style and finding meaning in one's life. The evolution of a postindustrial society brought with it the rise of a middle class seeking to improve their "quality of life" via professional services. The interest in and demand for hospice care was closely linked with this trend.

**Thanatologist: A New Profession**  Classical theory (Durkheim 1947) established that the division of labor was rooted in cultural survival. In an industrial society the demand was for goods and services that met basic needs such as food and shelter; work roles developed to meet these needs. Purpose or meaning was related to survival, and personal preference was not a driving force in one's choice of work role. In this classic paradigm, the owner of production was the person accorded high status.

Our postindustrial society, however, altered occupations and their status. As science and an industrial society improved the lives of the majority, a middle class emerged that demanded new services and professionals to provide such services. Many of these professionals (lawyers, accountants, counselors) and the services they provided had heretofore been available only to the upper class. Furthermore, as the production of goods could be accomplished by machines, work and work's value were redefined. In 1900 farm workers and laborers predominated; currently, professional and service workers make up the majority of the work force (Ritzer and Walczak 1986).

The public sought professionals' services, and in turn professionals encouraged the public to rely on their expertise. Physicians and lawyers were particularly successful in convincing the public that they had expert knowledge not easily understood (Freidson 1970a). Because of their expertise, these professions became self-regulated, and the autonomy, status, and financial benefits they achieved became goals for other occupational groups. Nurses, for example, have attempted to establish themselves as a profession independent of physicians' control.

The literature about the dying problem suggested that there was a need for a new kind of professional, a specialist, who would counterbalance the scientific, treatment-oriented tendencies of medical care. Schneidman (1973) described the need for clinical thanatologists to help people cope with death. Krant (1974) suggested that the thanatologist could function as a "human advocate in disease."

Because it was a new profession with no established training criteria or restrictions, people from various occupations entered this field. The professional brave enough to work with a dying person one week became an expert on the subject the following week (Kastenbaum and Costa 1977). Professionals seeking to improve their status by becoming experts in a new field—nurses, funeral directors, psychologists, and social workers—began calling themselves thanatologists.

Hospice programs created an egalitarian environment in which thanatologists could implement new practices designed to normalize dying, death, and grief. According to hospice philosophy, no one profession had special knowledge about death. Doctors, nurses, volunteers—all were considered to have expertise in the care of the dying. No team member, regardless of professional affiliation, was to dominate treatment decisions.

**The Search for Meaning** Participation in hospice programs also gave meaning to one's work. The search for a meaningful existence has become a common theme in Western civilization. Paloma (1982) summarized this search for meaning as a frustration that is part of modernity. "Modern culture has been accused of frustrating at least three basic human needs or desires: community, engagement, and dependence. Men and women are social beings and thus desire community. They seek meaning in life that is more than an extension of the ego—meaning that enables each to come to grips with personal and interpersonal problems. Furthermore, they seek dependence, which allows them to share responsibility for the direction of their lives" (35). As our postindustrial society freed people to pursue their own goals, not just labor to produce goods, the average person began to want more from employment than a paycheck, more from leisure than relaxation.

Traditional work takes place in large structures (bureaucracies) characterized by their emphasis on calculability, efficiency, predictability, and control (Weber, quoted in Miller 1971). Workers in these settings derive little benefit or pleasure from their role. "As tasks are divided and subdivided, it becomes increasingly difficult for workers to find satisfaction in the intrinsic aspects of their job" (Ritzer and Walczak 1986, 18). In hospital environments such bureaucratic characteristics are common, and they alienate staff because of the value placed on rules, routines, and paper procedures. Mechanic (1968), speaking of health care systems, stated that "social life generally is becoming more technically complicated, more differentiated, and more bureaucratized. There is a growing sense of loss of community, and social relationships are more segmented and less personalized" (11).

Hospice work provided something different. The work was not limited to accomplishing tasks, such as bathing, dressing, or medication review. Workers were encouraged to establish relationships with their charges. Caseloads were kept low so that staff could spend time talking with patients and families about their experiences, or just being a supportive presence. A staff of four might have as few as six to ten cases. This arrangement contrasted with the fragmented, poorly staffed, and task-oriented nature of health services in hospitals; health care workers, accustomed to large caseloads and inadequate support, found hospice programs a more desirable work environment. "Working toward good death is rewarding, and it is professionally fulfilling to support one another, especially in sharing burdens and pains brought to the surface as so often happens with death and human suffering" (Krant 1974, 97).

Participants also received help in coping with their feelings about their work. Hospice work, although rewarding, is stressful: workers face constant losses; patients do not get better, they die. Hospice leaders were concerned that staff would burn out without emotional support. Support groups were the most common vehicles for managing the emotions that come with the job. At these meetings, staff and volunteers were encouraged to discuss the feelings of loss and frustration that were constant themes in their work.

In the early phases of the movement, when there was little money to pay staff, there was no shortage of willing volunteers. These participants were ministers, physicians, nurses, social workers, funeral directors, lawyers, and psychologists, and they were willing to do whatever was necessary to make patient and family comfortable.

## Technological Progress and Its Consequences

For centuries medical scientists have attempted to eliminate infectious disease, extend life, treat degenerative disease, and reduce discomfort. Since the nineteenth century physicians have been designated the determiners of treatment and have had a professional monopoly over the health care system. Antibiotic treatments, reconstruction of damaged bones or blood vessels, and organ transplants are among the techniques that have reduced death and discomfort for numerous patients.

Although technological advances have enabled physicians to extend life, there are social consequences; people who live longer experience chronic degenerative diseases or, even worse, can survive in vegetative states. As scientific knowledge increased, to treat or not to treat became a theme in medical practice. Technology was painful as well as miraculous. Moreover, the ability to overcome some physical conditions has encouraged a belief that physicians can cure a myriad of physical and social problems that afflict human beings. The term *worried well* describes this new consumer of medical services.

Exploring the ability of medical science to extend life (or prolong the process of dying, as those opposed to such intervention would describe it) and cure disease is inherently problematic. Medical scientists' claims that they have vanquished disease are countered by researchers' assertions that medical science has had a limited effect on improving our health. Moreover, for as many advances as are made, there are concomitant problems. This section expands on those aspects of this topic that influenced the emergence and the claims of the hospice movement.

**Death: An Unnatural Event**  In the twentieth century death has been considered an insult to the scientific advance of medicine. According to Marcuse, people "experience death primarily as a technical limit of human freedom whose surpassing would become the recognized goal of individual and social endeavor" (1959, 69). If we look at mortality rates and the causes of death, we see that death from to acute illness, such as pneumonia or influenza, has been replaced by death from chronic degenerative disease, such as cancer and heart disease (see table 1).

**Table 1    The Ten Leading Causes of Death in the United States, 1900 and 1964**

| Rank | Cause of Death | Death Rate per 100,000 | % of Deaths from All Causes |
|---|---|---|---|
| | | **1900** | |
| 1 | Pneumonia and influenza | 202 | 11.8 |
| 2 | Tuberculosis | 194 | 11.3 |
| 3 | Diarrhea and enteritis | 143 | 8.3 |
| 4 | Diseases of the heart | 137 | 8.0 |
| 5 | Cerebral hemorrhage | 107 | 6.2 |
| 6 | Nephritis | 89 | 4.2 |
| 7 | Accidents | 72 | 4.2 |
| 8 | Cancer | 64 | 3.7 |
| 9 | Diphtheria | 40 | 2.3 |
| 10 | Meningitis | 34 | 2.0 |

Note: Represents 65% of total deaths; other causes unknown.

| Rank | Cause of Death | Death Rate per 100,000 | % of Deaths from All Causes |
|---|---|---|---|
| | | **1964** | |
| 1 | Diseases of the heart | 366 | 38.9 |
| 2 | Cancer and other malignancies | 151 | 16.1 |
| 3 | Cerebral hemorrhage | 104 | 11.0 |
| 4 | Accidents | 54 | 5.8 |
| 5 | Certain diseases of early infancy | 32 | 3.4 |
| 6 | Pneumonia and influenza (except of newborn) | 31 | 3.3 |
| 7 | General arteriosclerosis | 19 | 2.1 |
| 8 | Diabetes mellitus | 17 | 1.8 |
| 9 | Other diseases of circulatory system | 14 | 1.4 |
| 10 | Other bronchopulmonic diseases | 12 | 1.3 |

Note: Represents 85% total deaths; other causes include suicide, homicide, nephritis, etc.

Source: National Center for Health Statistics.

After the 1920s death took place in a sterile environment, the hospital, with the dying surrounded by specialists, not close family members. Estimates of the exact percentage of people who died in a place other than their home ranged from 70 percent to 90 percent (Fox 1979; Hefferman and Maynard 1977). Families supported medical treatments out of deference to technology and fear of guilt; seeking medical care reassured family members that everything possible was being done (Corbett and Hai 1979).

Technology that extended life, such as artificial respirators and organ transplants, increased the public's expectation that death before 90 years of age was an unnatural event. Cryonics, the process in which the body is frozen immediately after clinical death and then stored in liquid nitrogen, is the most extreme example of the lengths technology has gone to circumvent death. The procedure offers the possibility of being brought back to life at some point in the future when there is a treatment or cure for the person's cause of death.

The reliance on, and demand for, the best technology available, regardless of success rates, led to increased confusion about when active treatment should cease and when palliative care should begin. Hospice care provided one possible solution to this debate; it was a compromise that proposed using technology for comfort not cure, and it added another person's opinion, the patient's, to the process. Adapting technology to provide comfort rather than to extend life and allowing patients to participate in treatment decisions had the potential to alleviate physicians' responsibility for preserving life and their sense of failure when treatments were unsuccessful.

**The Discovery of New Drug Therapies**   During the 1950s and 1960s, when radiation and chemicals were new cancer treatments, they were associated with great physical discomfort and limited success. Harry, a man in his mid-50s, for example, was diagnosed as having metastatic disease. Despite a poor prognosis, he was placed on chemotherapy. At that time medical technology used strong doses of essentially poisonous material, injected at frequent intervals into the blood stream; the resultant nausea, vomiting, and discomfort had few sources of relief. Family and friends could only stand by and watch as Harry's condition slowly deteriorated, and they wondered if these treatments were worth the suffering. As such doubts gained public and professional attention during the 1960s, hospice care became a potential alternative to this troublesome scenario.

Advances in drug therapies also had their benefits. The discovery of a new way to administer drugs such as phenothiazines (tranquilizers) was consistent with Cicely Saunders's assertions about effective ways of administering barbiturates to control pain. Psychiatrists found that by establishing a stable dose of medication in the patient's blood stream they were better able to control his or her psychiatric symptoms. Saunders suggested a similar use of barbiturates; instead of waiting for pain to occur, staff should administer barbiturates to cancer patients around the clock to prevent symptoms for starting. Once pain began, Saunders asserted, it was harder to control and required larger doses of barbiturates.

The discovery of medications to reduce psychiatric symptoms and appropriate ways to administer them did not directly result in physicians employing round-the-clock techniques when prescribing barbiturates. It did, however, produce a willing group of physicians, psychiatrists, who understood pain management techniques and were willing to use them. Early hospice providers turned to psychiatrists to act as medical directors and oversee drug therapies that had not yet become part of mainstream medical practice.

**Critics of Technology's Claims** Countering the expansion and praise of modern health care were those who asserted that medical science's gains were overstated. Dubos (1959) was one of the first to point this out. He stated that many factors other than medical technology were responsible for improved survival rates: "But while modern science can boast of so many startling achievements in the health fields, its role has not been so unique and its effectiveness not so complete as is commonly claimed. By the time laboratory medicine came effectively into the picture the job had been carried far toward completion by the humanitarians and social reformers of the nineteenth century. . . . When the tide is receding from the beach it is easy to have the illusion that one can empty the ocean by removing water with a pail. The tide of infectious and nutritional diseases was rapidly receding when the laboratory scientist moved into action at the end of the past century" (22–23).

Claims that treatments for cancer patients had dramatically raised cure rates were also questioned. Epstein (1978) asserted that the ability to survive surgery explained increased cancer survival. The modest improvements in cancer cure rates achieved from the 1930s to the 1950s were the result of better surgical techniques and postoperative procedures, critics argued, rather than early detection or cure as the result of new drug therapies. "For a majority of the 12 most common tumors there was little or no improvement from 1950 to 1982 in the rate that patients survived their disease" (Boffey 1987, A1).

Harsh attacks on contemporary medical treatments have become more common. Peele (1989), who believes that improved community supports, not treatments, are needed, stated: "Even in the case of cancer, we have remained stuck in our tendency to invest massively in frontal attacks against disease agents and mechanisms. Since 1971 when Congress declared an official war on cancer, we have exponentially increased our investment in finding the cause and cure for disease. Almost twenty years later, having now spent billions of dollars, this attack has produced few benefits and no cures" (9).

Diagnostic methods had not reduced cancer illness, but they had improved physicians' ability to detect disease processes. As doctors were able to diagnose cancer at earlier stages, survival times increased, but the statistical method for categorizing cancer sufferers cured remained the same. Consequently, survival rates increased because methods of data collection were unchanged, not because diseases were cured.

Illich (1976) observed physician practice during the 1950s and declared that health care had become depersonalized. Instead of physicians treating patients, they put them in beds and treated their charts. Furthermore, he asserted that medical treatments were as much a source of disease as they were a cure. Iatrogenic diseases, illnesses caused by medical treatments, were common, substituting one disease for another. When some members of society heard these claims, they rejected traditional medical practice and sought alternatives, including holistic health care and nontraditional cancer treatments such as laetrile.

Early leaders of the hospice movement took such critics seriously. They believed that science's curative abilities were overrated and that for many terminally ill patients treatment increased discomfort. They also believed, however, that health care could be altered to provide comfort. For example, instead of putting a feeding tube into a patient's stomach, a volunteer could slowly spoon-feed liquids, thus preventing the patient from being starved or dehydrated but doing so in a less invasive way. As hospice providers became part of the health care system, however, their ability to separate treatment for comfort and treatment for cure diminished. Furthermore, participation in medical systems encouraged an emphasis on treatment routines; hand-holding and other forms of comfort were lesser priorities.

**Physician Dominance and Consumer Demands** Consistent with assertions that medical science was unable to accomplish all of its claims were criticisms of consumers' overuse of physicians and physicians' control over health care. The twentieth-century consumer of medical care expects physicians to ameliorate pain and suffering. "As a nation we seem particularly vulnerable to the expertise of professionals. This is perhaps part of the belief that all things in life can be reduced to logical parameters" (Krant 1974, 11). For the most part, people trust that their doctors know more about how they feel than they themselves do. "We have turned our bodies over to the physician with little control over the profession which deems treatment" (Friedson 1970a, 83). One consequence of physicians' autonomy has been that physicians make decisions for patients, not with them. Surveys of physicians (Weir 1986) found that doctors don't feel obliged to tell their patients about their diseases. Such practices aroused ethicists' interest, and they questioned physicians' right to withhold information from patients.

By the 1960s, when the hospice movement emerged, scholars had identified physician dominance over treatment, and some consumers had begun to seek alternative methods of treatment. Efforts to reform health care, however, had not reached the stage of collective action, and the hospice movement did not attempt to politicize the issue. The lack of consumer opposition to the general health care system influenced consumers' to hospice care. Most did not demand hospice services, nor did they request control over their medical treatments. Without the support for change from consumers, reformers had difficulty achieving their goals.

The formation of coalitions by AIDS activists to combat traditional health care practices is an unusual example of health care consumers fighting the system. Discrimination in access to health care services and lack of speedy approval processes for new treatments are among the issues that groups such as Act Up have addressed. Along with bringing attention to such practices, their efforts have resulted in faster approval processes for some AIDS treatments.

**Ethics** Scientific discoveries increased treatment options and outcomes. As alternatives became available decisions about treatment became more complicated, and ethicists debated the consequences of technology. Ethical concerns were shared by the medical community, and physicians pondered bioethical issues. The medical profession's concern for the consequences of science illuminates the complexity of the conditions under which hospice care became popular. Although the medical profession was accused of promoting aggressive treatments, the same profession was willing to question its practices.

A major factor in the dispute regarding the wisdom of using medical technology to preserve life (or prolong dying) was the increase in people who survived in vegetative states—conditions where vital organs function but the individual is not alert or able to communicate. Medical technology had advanced to the point that machines were able to compensate for an ailing organ, such as the heart or lung. For some, this technology served a life-saving function while an organ healed, but for others it extended life despite irreparable brain damage. Extension of life was less desirable when it meant survival of the body without perceivable participation in life. As medical science developed life-supporting technology, physicians and families had to decide when hope of recovery should be given up and when withdrawal of the technology constituted murder.

Recent advances in the treatment of severe head trauma, for example, increased survival rates, but as the following case shows, those who survived did not always resume full functioning. Joe was a 25-year-old male who had suffered a head injury in a street fight. Technological advances maintained life support systems while surgery reduced massive internal bleeding, but not before extensive, irreversible brain damage had occurred. Joe was no longer conscious or able to communicate by word or gesture that he was cognizant of his surroundings. After several months he no longer required acute care, and he was placed in a nursing home.

Keeping Joe alive meant preventing infections from developing by monitoring the various tubes that fed and cleansed his body. A person who is incapable of movement is prone to systemic infections, which, if permitted to persist, would ultimately result in death. In America, biological treatments are commonplace; nonaggressive and supportive (palliative) care include the use of intravenous antibiotics to prevent death. This meant someone as young as Joe could be kept alive for several years, despite the fact that there was no hope of improvement.

Members of the clergy were among the first to support patient and family rights to request that under certain circumstances treatment should cease, and they established procedures for making such decisions. In 1957 Pope Pius XII distinguished ordinary from extraordinary means of supporting life, stating that in certain situations extraordinary means should not be continued. He defined "extraordinary" as whatever was obtained through excessive expense, pain, and other inconvenience for the patient or for others. Furthermore, those treatments would not offer a reasonable hope or benefit to the patient (Saunders 1976). The church's position has remained consistent since the 1950s, and pastoral caregivers have supported family members who seek legal recourse to have medical treatments stopped.

The Catholic church also supported the hospice movement. During the mid-1970s, when hospice leaders wanted the medical community's support, the Catholic Hospital Association (CHA) reaffirmed its commitment to special services for dying patients. "The CHA board resolved on Nov 7, 1977, that the concept of the Catholic Hospice service was an integral part of the contemporary healing ministry, and voted that CHA should offer encouragement, consultation and other assistance to support establishment of this service by the association's constituent members and their sponsoring organizations" (Spillane 1979, 47).

**Euthanasia** The ability to support life that is essentially vegetative captured the attention of the public as it witnessed families who suffered the emotional, social, and financial consequences of preserving the life of a chronically ill relative. One response, albeit a controversial one, was euthanasia, or mercy killing. Euthanasia, like suicide, is largely disapproved of in Western civilization; it is incompatible with the values of the culture's established institutions. The belief in physicians' ability to cure makes any effort toward cessation of treatment even more difficult (Feifel 1977b). The debate about euthanasia is longstanding, but in the 1960s attention to this issue increased.

Euthanasia is typically categorized as active or passive. Active euthanasia, as the term suggests, is any act that deliberately shortens a terminally ill person's life. Someone takes the person's life with a drug or lethal weapon, or someone supplies the dying person with the means to take his or her own life. Passive euthanasia condones practices that result in natural death. The most common method of passive euthanasia is the cessation of artificial life-support systems.

In some more primitive cultures mercy killing is commonplace.[2] Complex societies have typically forbidden such practices, but certain elements of the society have always supported it. Greeks, for example, forbade suicide and mercy killing, but certain philosophers accepted the idea of ending a meaningless life. Greek physicians sought to preserve life, but "Aristotle and Plato endorsed infanticide as a means of ensuring the worthiest state for the worthiest individuals" (Humphry and Wickett 1986, 3).

The rise of Christianity strengthened opposition to active and passive euthanasia, and it was not until the Renaissance that certain factions again supported euthanasia. "Efforts to keep patients alive often caused suffering, which threatened to diminish the value of life. Bacon, Montaigne, More, and Donne were among the first to demand a merciful release from the new 'technology' of their times" (Humphry and Wickett 1986, 9). Disgrace awaited the surviving family of those who did choose to end their lives. People who committed suicide were not given a proper burial, and their possessions were confiscated by the state. By the eighteenth century, however, perpetrating indignities on the body of a suicide or burying it in an unholy grave were infrequent practices.

During the nineteenth century, some physicians became advocates of mercy killing.

> A handful of doctors wrote and spoke about suicide and the dying patient. Didn't every patient deserve to die "well"? In 1869 William Lecky referred to euthanasia as an act of "inducing an easy death." In 1889, while speaking to the Maine Medical Association, Dr. Frank E. Hitchcock urged physicians not to ignore the needs of terminally ill patients, especially those in pain Such suffering should be relieved, he argued; ultimately, fairness and justice "would regard the intent of the physician who humanely assists the patient in and out of his suffering." (Humphry and Wickett 1986, 11)

The first documented court case, which became the precedent for prosecuting mercy killings, occurred in Massachusetts in 1816. A prisoner in the cell next to a condemned man encouraged this second prisoner to end his life and thus cheat the waiting crowd from witnessing his hanging. The condemned man hung himself, and the first prisoner was charged with murder. The prosecution of this case was based on the question of whether anyone had the right to encourage death prematurely, regardless of how imminent death was (Beavan 1959). Although the law defined the action as murderous, the jury acquitted him.

Surveys of physicians in the twentieth century showed that most routinely accelerated the dying process or withheld treatments that would prolong life. For example, a surgeon who upon performing surgery found that a patient had incurable cancer might leave an open vein, known as a bleeder, and administer barbiturates so that the person would feel no discomfort. The patient soon died from internal bleeding. Another way that physicians hastened death was by administering large doses of barbiturates or by withholding antibiotic treatments.

Social Darwinism introduced another facet to the practice of euthanasia; should the feeble or less capable members of society be maintained by those who are better functioning? As early as 1895 it was suggested that the state allow physicians to kill feeble or degenerate infants by administering morphine. Although no official policy permitting such a procedure was ever established, informally such practices occurred. Infants born with serious congenital defects were allowed to die of starvation or, in some cases, were chloroformed (Dempsey 1975).

The memory of what occurred in Nazi Germany is a major argument against legitimating any form of euthanasia (Lautner and Meyer 1984). In 1933 the National Socialist party initiated phase one of their eugenic practices. They sterilized the mentally and physically impaired and then instituted phase two, "the children action," which was the annihilation, without family permission or knowledge, of those children deemed unnecessary or of no value. The third part of their plan mandated "mercy" killings of all those considered incurably sick; this included the developmentally disabled and mentally ill. Finally, they embarked on the genocide of Jews, prostitutes, homosexuals, and anyone viewed as a threat to the future of the Third Reich. They justified their activities as necessary to purify the world of undesirable traits.

Consequently, attempts to legalize passive or active euthanasia have been unsuccessful in most Western cultures. Bills to legalize euthanasia have been introduced repeatedly in Great Britain's House of Lords, but they have not been passed. Groups such as the Euthanasia Society, begun in England in 1936 and in America in 1938, attempted to gain popular support for this concept, but their efforts have been countered by such groups as the Human Rights Society, which supports preserving life regardless of a person's functional ability.

The right to expedite the dying process continues to be officially viewed as illegal, but perpetrators typically are not treated harshly. A random review of cases reported in the *New York Times* from 1959 to 1990 reflects the differential treatment of individuals who actively seek to end others' lives. Spouses, siblings, and parents of terminally ill patients who took their relative's life were consistently tried as murderers, but the family member was acquitted of the charges or granted early release from prison.

Physicians were also prosecuted for misusing medical treatments to shorten terminally ill patients' lives. They, too, were acquitted but only after a more protracted period of investigation. The now well-known Michigan physician Jack Kevorkian publicized the issue of physician-assisted death after using a "suicide machine" he developed to assist in the suicide of two women with Alzheimer's disease in 1992. Charges of murder were brought against him and then dismissed. He has repeatedly asserted that physicians have the responsibility to alleviate suffering of the terminally ill through assisted suicide. Health care professionals who have assumed responsibility for ending a number of lives without patient consent, however, have been unlikely candidates for acquittal.

Public opinion has increasingly favored mercy killings. In 1950 a Gallup poll found that 36 percent of the population sampled supported mercy killing for the incurably ill, and by 1973, 53 percent supported such practices. Robert Veatch researched proposed legislation regarding euthanasia in the 1960s and found that 40 separate bills had been introduced to legalize one or another aspect of euthanasia (Fulton and Owen 1981).

Advocates of passive euthanasia have until recently had little political success. Nancy Cruzan, a young woman from Missouri who became comatose after being in an automobile accident, is an example of the difficulty that families may experience when trying to cease life support systems and of the growing influence of right-to-life groups. Three years after the accident she did not show the slightest signs of improvement, and her parents asked to have the feeding tubes that kept her alive removed. Without Nancy's consent physicians were uncomfortable ending treatment, and the state attorney's office was asked to rule on the case.

The lack of a national policy regarding the "right to die" and the political influence of right-to-life interest groups resulted in decisions being made on a case-by-case basis after protracted periods of litigation. In Nancy's case the family's request to cease treatment led to a four-year court battle to determine if Nancy would have wanted to die. The debate was complicated by the assertions of some right-to-life advocates that removing the feeding tubes constituted murder. Finally, in December 1990, the court agreed that the tubes should be removed. Nancy died 12 days later.

Exit, a British group, and the Hemlock Society, located in California, advocate legalization of active euthanasia and help terminally ill patients commit suicide by providing instructions as to the most effective methods. Derek Humphry's recent best-seller, *Final Exit,* was first published in the 1970s but became popular only after its re-release in the early 1990s. Attempts to legalize euthanasia continue. Proposition 161, on the ballot in California in 1992, proposed that terminally ill patients with a six-month prognosis and the recommendation of two physicians be allowed to request a lethal dose of barbituates.

One development that has attracted attention to the practice of active euthanasia is the rise of AIDS sufferers. Particularly in the gay community, persons with AIDS have committed suicide when they believed that the disease had reached a stage where survival would mean only protracted suffering and no hope of remission. AIDS victims who want to end their lives often receive guidance and support to ingest or inject a lethal dose of barbiturates. This practice is called "assisted death," because the PWA usually involves family and friends in the act of taking the overdose and ending his or her life. When right-to-life advocates heard of two assisted deaths that took place in California, they attempted to prosecute those who had participated. Criminal proceedings in these cases were dropped. Although right-to-life advocates continue to pursue legal recourse to stop such activities, many more people have engaged in them.

The Catholic church has supported families' requests to cease treatments under extraordinary circumstances and has thus encouraged the spread of hospice programs, but the Church opposes any practice that actively brings about death. Cardinal Bernadin in Chicago called for Catholic cooperation in opposing active euthanasia, and Cardinal O'Connor of New York in 1989 suggested the establishment of an order of nuns, The Sisters of Life, to work against abortion and active euthanasia.

The debate over whether certain kinds of mercy killing should be allowed and over who should make that decision heated up during the late 1960s. Hospice care was a middle ground between allowing someone to die without any treatment and using every machine and method possible to delay death, even if the patient had no hope of recovery. Hospice leaders avowed that their emphasis was on living, not dying, but some people still saw hospice care as another form of mercy killing. At times such views resulted in failed attempts by hospice groups to institute programs or in the refusal of private physicians to refer patients to hospice care.

Of all the social conditions that influenced the hospice movement's development, it was the practice of euthanasia that elicited the greatest opposition from hospice advocates. Early in the movement's history leaders vehemently opposed euthanasia and asserted that hospice was not a form of mercy killing. Advocates of hospice care argued that its emphasis on healing and treating suffering often eliminated the patient's desire to end life. According to Cicely Saunders (1976), a patient's request to die often reflects a wish to end suffering; patients that are treated properly may live longer and without discomfort.

To summarize, the ability to determine when natural death will occur continues to elude scientists. Who lives and who dies often is at odds with medical interventions; the patient with the best prognosis may die from other complications. Still, dependence on machines and the suspicion that the failure to use aggressive treatment cheats the person of prolonged life continue to dominate health care.

## Terminal Care Costs

As care of the sick in the United States changed from familial to organizational systems and the demand for technology increased, the cost of care increased. Scientists focused on improving technology to cure disease, but health care managers concerned themselves with containing costs. Policymakers called this latter process "rational managed care."

All the previously described factors were important in attracting a broad base of popular support for the hospice movement. Research about death's psychological and sociological impact and new treatments for dying patients made the concept of hospice care more popular, but it was the movement's willingness to reduce the cost of care that made it attractive to third-party reimbursers and legitimized it as an alternative to acute health care.

**Health Care Costs**  Estimates of the increase in medical costs range from 10 percent to 20 percent per year. These figures far outstrip the national inflation rate, and health care costs take an increasingly large chunk out of the gross national product. In 1974 health care costs were $1.4 trillion, or 9 percent of the GNP, by 1990 they had reached 12 percent, and in the year 2000 they are expected to reach 15 percent of GNP. Furthermore, about 20 percent to 30 percent of health care dollars are expended on care of terminally ill patients (Veatch 1988). The rise of health care costs are attributed to use of services, few price controls, and rapid technological change.

**The Expanding Health Care Industry**  The ability to prolong life has increased the number of people who survive with chronic degenerative conditions, thus increasing morbidity rates while decreasing mortality rates. As these chronic degenerative conditions were redefined as illnesses, they required treatment by health care providers (Strauss and Corbin 1988). Physicians encouraged those labeled sick to turn themselves over to technicians' care in specialized settings. Chronic conditions, however, require intermittent rather than constant care, so alternatives to the acute health care system were needed. Nursing facilities and home health agencies developed to accommodate the changing nature of health care. As extensions of the acute health care system, such agencies maintained the chronically ill person in their sick role until physicians' attentions were needed or until patients were designated cured. Creating these new services also served to expand the health care industry. Policymakers assumed that such expansion would lower health care costs because it substituted less expensive services for costly, acute care services. But the new programs consistently raised rather than reduced costs (Hoyer 1990).

Prior to the introduction of hospice services, terminally ill patients posed a problem for health care providers. Nursing homes and home care services were unable to manage dying patients' needs, families were reluctant to assume home care responsibilities, and physicians were therefore forced to maintain dying patients in expensive hospital beds. (Compounding the family's reluctance to care for the dying was the changed role of women. After the 1950s, more women entered the work force, and they were therefore less available to care for chronically sick family members.) Hospice care was attractive to policymakers because of its potential for containing terminal care costs. Yet, based on their experience funding nursing homes and end-stage renal disease, policymakers had reservations about alternative systems' capacity to fulfill this potential. Consequently, support for hospice care was mixed.

**Cost-Containing Efforts** Efforts to curb medical costs in the United States began to develop in the 1950s as new equipment and increased morbidity escalated the use of medical services. Policymakers sought ways to reduce health care costs while maintaining access to, and quality of, services. Considering the likelihood of a procedure's success and examining subjective factors such as age or work history were some of the ways that policymakers attempted to decide who should or should not receive treatment. For example, in England, where there is greater tolerance for restricting access to health care, the determination of who receives intensive rehabilitation is based on factors such as age, previous work history, contribution to society, and potential for recovery (Halper 1987).

In the United States, policies about access to services are determined in a less consistent fashion. Age is one factor used to determine who receives aggressive treatment. The young mother will receive the latest available technology even when there is limited probability of success; the 85-year-old grandmother will have less difficulty encouraging physicians to cease and desist. But if an elderly person wants a procedure and can pay for it, he or she can usually find a physician and hospital that will perform the requested service.

Social status, although a subjective measure, is the most common determinant of who receives treatment. This is partly because of the low value we place on certain groups of people and because the tab for such expenditures is picked up by the public welfare system—a system that is usually short of sufficient funds to pay for all the services requested of it. For example, studies have shown that minorities or people perceived as being of low status (street people, alcoholics) were less likely to receive the best life-saving techniques available. Research on the way that a lay citizen panel determined renal transplant recipients in Washington state found that "Henry David Thoreau would have a poor chance of being approved for a kidney transplant by this committee" (Dempsey 1975, 29).

In response to the increased need for chronic care, reimbursement structures for long-term care, such as nursing home or home care services, were instituted under the Medicare and Medicaid programs in 1967. Although developed to curb costs, new services increased expenditures. Statistics on nursing home growth from 1954 to 1969, for example, indicated that reimbursement encouraged expansion of the nursing home industry rather than a reduction in acute health care use. In 1954 there were only 6,539 nursing homes in America; by 1969 the number had doubled to 13,047 (Monroe 1973). Almost as soon as policymakers started paying for nursing home care, they also looked for ways to restrict access to government-funded, long-term care. The establishment of coverage for end-stage renal disease had similar financial consequences (Aiken and Marx 1982).

Research indicated that a significant proportion of health care dollars was spent during the last year of life (Buckingham 1982–83); hospice care, with its low emphasis on treatments and inpatient services, presented a way to provide cheaper terminal care. Concurrently, once the first programs were created, hospice advocates turned their attention to acquiring national funding for hospice services. When they recognized cost-effectiveness was important to policymakers, hospice leaders set out to prove the cost benefits of their services.

At the time hospice care was being considered for reimbursement, however, policymakers were becoming skeptical of funding new programs. Leaders of the hospice movement had to accept severe funding restrictions in return for eligibility for public funds. Policymakers established caps and limitations on inpatient services, thus assuring that patients opting for hospice care would save the government money. Furthermore, reimbursements were provided for those aspects of hospice programs that were in keeping with the traditional health care system and were low in cost, such as in-home nursing services; inpatient care, which is the most expensive service, was severely restricted. Funding restrictions influenced hospice programs, particularly programs created after Medicare regulations were established. Said differently, after Medicare established its guidelines, hospice programs' form was shaped by funding, not the ideals of the movement.

## Conclusion

The popular belief in the 1960s that we had become a death-denying society paved the way for the hospice movement. The ability of hospice programs to meet the social and psychological needs of participants while adding a new service made such programs compatible with the dominant trend of the time, an expanding health care industry. As providers' claims that hospice care could ease death's pains and cut costs became accepted truths, the rise of the movement and the spread of programs was assured, but at a cost to the movement's ideals.

*Chapter 4*

# Death with Dignity and the Emergence of the Hospice Movement

Tracing the origins of the hospice movement is difficult. During the incipient stage of any social movement organized efforts to change social beliefs or practices are absent; instead, vague, unconnected incidents suggest an emerging interest. The incipient stage of the hospice movement was further obscured by the fact that it did not begin as a separate social cause but as part of another social movement—death with dignity. To depict the hospice movement's incipience, we must first trace the rise of the death with dignity movement.

During the 1950s and 1960s "good death," or death with dignity, became popular among social scientists and humanitarians. The death with dignity movement arose from the belief that death in American culture was denied. For a time, there was little to distinguish members of the hospice movement from members of the death with dignity movement. People who were interested in these issues interacted in a variety of activities designed to promote "good death" and were loosely unified by an organization called the International Work Group on Death, Dying, and Bereavement (IWG). The formation of the Yale Study Group in 1967 marked the separation of the hospice and death with dignity movements, although interaction between the members of the two groups persisted.

The hospice movement shared with the death with dignity movement a desire to return control of the dying process to the individual. But it also sought to offer comfort through the use of innovative medical treatments. These twin goals—one aiming for less involvement from the medical community, the other requiring more—were incompatible. Consequently, neither would ever be fully achieved.

## Death with Dignity: An Obscure Social Movement

Several scholars have described the collective activities aimed at ameliorating conditions for the dying. In 1977 Hefferman and Maynard stated, "The public concern about the plight of the dying has picked up in recent years. The movement promoting this issue as a social problem is just getting started. The movement is only in the early stage of rise (incipiency or close to coalescence), and is not yet moving fast" (101). Strauss, writing in 1975, corroborated the existence of the movement: "Since the middle 1960s the concern with proper and more humanistic dying has mounted steadily, principally perhaps, among non-physician health workers and religious personnel" (196). In 1978 Kastenbaum called it a "death awareness" movement, and Fox acknowledged the evolution of a "death with dignity" movement in 1979, citing Elisabeth Kübler-Ross as its charismatic leader.

Besides these scholarly references, research and written descriptions of the death with dignity movement are sparse. Public awareness and documentation of social movements vary. Some attempts at social reform, such as prohibition or women's suffrage, receive so much attention and are such integral components of our cultural history that they are common knowledge; other movements are remembered by only a few. The Townsend movement (Fisher 1978), for example, tried to establish a retirement savings program before Roosevelt's New Deal reforms. Although popular during the 1930s and 1940s, the Townsend movement is now known to only a few scholars. The death with dignity movement appears to be destined to a similar, obscure place in history.

The organizations that made up the death with dignity movement never created a legitimizing body or authoritarian base from which to institutionalize their ideas. Without such formal efforts to bring about change, any impact that these groups had on society was idiosyncratic and not identified as part of a social movement. The inability to claim accomplishments, such as a program or policy, would limit popular attention and interest in chronicling the movement's history.

For example, the popularization of self-help groups for the bereaved can be attributed to the death with dignity movement. Groups for grieving spouses and family members exist nationwide and are held in churches and community agencies. They are not nationally organized, and there are no formal policies mandating their existence; the issue was never politicized and no effort was made to institutionalize bereavement groups. Bereavement groups exist because the death with dignity movement made people sensitive to the needs of grieving people, and humanitarians came forward to assist survivors.

Another problem with describing this movement is its association with the hospice movement, which has often created the impression that the two were one. Those directly involved in the death with dignity movement are quick to distinguish themselves from the hospice movement. They describe the hospice movement not as the *sine qua non* of their activities but as one way to provide care to terminally ill patients.

"Hospice was made into a big thing, but it was really just a way to meet a need," stated Elizabeth Pritchard, an assistant professor at Columbia University's College of Physicians and Surgeons and a member of the Foundation of Thanatology (personal communication). She viewed hospice as a way to provide care for the increasing number of terminally ill patients. Other core members agree. They report that the major interest among the death with dignity movement's participants was to understand the process of grieving, to bring death and dying out of the closet, and to establish patient controls over the health care process.

The hospice movement also differed from the death with dignity movement in its constituents. Descriptions of the hospice movement characterize it as a people's movement or a grass roots reform effort: "Increasing public concern with quality of life of the dying patient has resulted in efforts to improve medical care" (Hays and Arnold 1986, 130). Had the hospice movement remained part of the death with dignity movement this description would be accurate. Participants in the hospice movement, however, were primarily health care workers who were dissatisfied with the general standards of care for dying patients; the lay public had little input into the political processes or goals of the hospice movement.

**Death: An Emerging Social Problem** During the 1950s and 1960s death became more than just an event in the life cycle, "death became fashionable" (Dempsey 1975). The writings and activities of these two decades provide evidence of a growing interest in thanatology, particularly the consequences of grief, dying, and death on patients and survivors. Moreover, activities during the 1950s, such as the organization of conferences and the formation of agencies, indicate that the dying process had become an acknowledged social problem. During the next decade the dying problem became popular, people were openly disgruntled by cultural attitudes and behaviors toward dying people and their survivors, and formal groups assembled to reform cultural practices.

Herman Feifel's *The Meaning of Death,* an anthology of psychological and philosophical writings on death in Western culture published in 1959, is the best remembered work of the 1950s. Hospice leaders cite Feifel's book as the inspiration for the hospice movement. Social scientists, health care workers, and the public read it and were motivated to reexamine their perceptions of treatment for the dying and to seek out other individuals similarly disposed. Other scholars, such as John Hinton and Collin Murray Parkes, also studied death's social and psychological impact and helped raise public and professional consciousness about this issue.

Clinicians attracted to this topic were particularly concerned with death's psychological impact. Some helped health care workers talk about their concerns regarding dying patients and their families, and others recommended intervention strategies to reduce the stress experienced by patient and family (Eissler 1955; Ogg 1959). Nurse educators encouraged professionals to examine their tendency to provide adequate physical care but to avoid patients' attempts to talk about death and dying. Mental health workers recognized that their clients needed special care to cope with death and dying, and they developed educational and supportive services to amend this situation.

One American pioneer in bringing death and dying out of the closet was Esther L. Brown, a nurse educator. In 1952 she asked a group of health care workers if they would like to do something to help comfort terminally ill patients or if they felt this responsibility fell to the clergy. Following her lecture an attendee drew her aside to ask what could be done. Brown suggested that a group of health care workers or community members might be willing to assemble and discuss the issue. The nurse posing the question was unable to imagine that anyone other than the chaplain would join such a group. Brown found that the views expressed by this nurse were shared by others in the nursing profession, leading her to include in her workshops for nursing staff discussions about the physical and emotional needs of dying patients and their families (National Conference on Social Welfare, 1978).

Two events in England also indicated a changing attitude toward death and dying. First, in the 1950s, the Madame Curie Foundation found that more hospice programs were needed to help families cope with terminal illness. "The provision of residential homes," the foundation reported, "would save much mental suffering, stress, and strain for relatives" (Lamerton 1975, 154). Consequently, 12 homes in the British Isles were opened strictly for the care of cancer patients (Downie 1973). Second, Cicely Saunders became the first medical officer at Saint Joseph's hospice. "She came to Saint Joseph's with a conviction that pain for the dying was unnecessary, and set out to prove it" (Lamerton 1975, 154). Saunders publicized her accomplishments in a series of articles for the British journal *Nursing Times*. Her methods emphasized "the Christian imperative to offer healing whether that be easing pain so the person can get better or allowing death when its time has come" (Saunders 1976, 6).

Back in America, recognition that health care in hospitals was not sufficient for those suffering chronic degenerative illness resulted in the establishment of new programs to help patients and families. Two medical social workers, working in acute care hospitals in New York City, were concerned about the lack of available services for patients once they were discharged, and they appealed to the National Cancer Foundation for financial support to create a nonprofit voluntary agency. This agency, Cancer Care, continues to provide free counseling services for cancer patients and their families in New York City. The American Cancer Society also responded to the rising demand for supportive services. Traditionally, funds had been allocated to medical research, but as social workers made the agency aware of patient and family needs, it earmarked funds to be used for psychosocial support.

National conferences held during this decade also served to spread the word. The National Cancer Foundation sponsored "A Symposium on Terminal Illness" in 1956 and "A Constructive Approach to Terminal Illness" in 1958. Help for dying patients and their families was not the exclusive interest of cancer care providers. In 1956 Herman Feifel held the first session on death and dying at the Annual Meeting of the American Psychological Association, and in 1959 the National Conference on Social Welfare had its first session on social work intervention with dying patients and their families.

**The Death with Dignity Movement Coalesces**  As the death with dignity movement's cause became popular in the 1960s and 1970s, groups assembled in hospitals, parishes, and colleges to talk about ways to change social conditions. Assemblies such as these served to reinforce participants' belief that something was wrong with the way the dying were treated and that social reform was required. Their point of departure for any discussion was that America was a death-denying culture and that the dying and their survivors were consequently not allowed to acknowledge their pain and suffering. The exchange of ideas provided the emotional impetus necessary to propel the death with dignity movement forward; informal interest was transformed into formal organization.

The ideas espoused by the death with dignity movement were politicized in the 1970s when the Senate heard testimony on the plight of the dying. "The changing attitude toward aspects of death and dying following Kübler-Ross was epitomized by the Senate hearing on 'Death with Dignity' in August, 1972. Among the topics considered at this hearing were the right to die, living-will legislation, the legal definition of death, the increasing technology of health care systems, and the plans and hopes for hospice care in the United States" (Rinaldi and Kearl 1990, 285–86).

The proliferation of scholarly references further attests to the rising interest in thanatology. In 1964 Robert Fulton found only 400 citations for a bibliography on this subject; by 1977 he could list 3,800 titles (Fulton 1977). Organizations were also created to conduct research and distribute information. Among them were the Center for Death Education and Research at the University of Minnesota, the Foundation of Thanatology in New York, the Continental Association of Funeral and Memorial Services in Washington, D.C., the National Funeral Directors Association in Milwaukee, Equinox in Boston, and Ars Moriendi in Philadelphia. Robert Fulton, Austin Kutscher, and Robert Kastenbaum were among the leaders who developed and directed these organizations.

As a result of bioethical debates in the 1970s, moratoriums were called on certain procedures, such as heart transplants, psychosurgery, fetal surgery, and in-vitro fertilization. Concerns were raised that patients were being offered treatments with little hope of success; the patient served to advance the course of medical science at the expense of his or her quality of life and the family's peace of mind (Fox 1979). To promote discussion of medical ethics, Drs. Robert Veatch and Willard Gaylin formed the Institute of Society, Ethics, and Life Sciences as part of the Columbia College of Physicians. In their first year they received 29 requests from medical schools to speak about this topic (Fox 1979).

Organizations such as these came about not only through the efforts of enlightened intellectuals who were aware of research about death denial; personal experience also played a part. Austin Kutscher was a physician who through his own grief experience recognized that society lacked information about death's emotional impact. Following the death of his first wife he found little support or information available to help him cope with, or understand, his feelings of grief. He decided to create a foundation to promote scientific investigation into these issues, and in 1966 formed the Foundation of Thanatology.

The foundation is also an example of the way hospice advocates participated in organizational activities of the death with dignity movement. Kutscher started it to promote medical research on death, dying, and grief. Among the participants at its symposiums were Dr. Samuel Klagsbrun and Rev. Carlton Sweetser, who lectured about hospice care as one way to ameliorate conditions for the dying and who became leaders in the hospice movement.

As organizations sprang up and information increased, thanatologists created publications specifically devoted to death and dying. In 1966 Robert Kastenbaum and Richard Kalish published the first of these, a newsletter. In 1970 this newsletter became the journal *Omega*. The first edition of the *Hastings Center Reports*, a journal put out by a bioethical research institute of the same name, was published in 1969. As the director of the institute stated, "We were nothing at that point but a small group of people with an idea that the emerging ethical problems of medicine and biology deserved some serious and sustained attention" (Callahan 1979). *Death Studies* was another journal developed during the 1970s, to accommodate the proliferation of research on this topic.

As the leaders of the death with dignity movement gathered followers, the relatively small, intimate meetings of the 1960s were replaced by large symposia and college seminars. The first significant symposium was held in 1970 at Hamline University in Saint Paul, Minnesota. More than 2,000 people attended (Feifel 1977a). Efforts to institutionalize teaching about death, dying, and grief peaked during the 1970s. Fulton (1977) reported that 2,000 new thanatology courses were offered at the college and university level in the years 1974–77.

**The Movement's Accomplishments**   The death with dignity movement opposed several social institutions and their practices. First were the hospitals, where dying people were isolated and where the staff ignored their emotional needs. Next were various social institutions (churches, schools, and workplaces) that did not tolerate free expressions of grief. Another was the mortuary system, which cosmeticized death and made it expensive but did little to ease survivors' grief. The movement's opposition to these institutions and practices was often ad hoc rather than organized, and this makes its accomplishments difficult to measure. Humanistic, normalizing practices were intertwined with new medical treatments. As Krant suggested, "Terms such as death with dignity are often heard, but the art and manner of its accomplishment are poorly reckoned" (1974, 97). The following sections describe a few outcomes of the movement's efforts to ameliorate conditions for the dying and their survivors.

*Normalizing Grief* Phyllis Silverman, a social worker, advocated demedicalizing and normalizing the grieving process. Silverman conceptualized grief as a life passage, not a pathological process, and she suggested that people who had gone through this process were in the best position to help others. To test her ideas, she designed the widow-to-widow project at Harvard Medical School. This project began in 1967 and extended through 1973. Widows who had been through the grieving process were asked to reach out to recent widows, who were then given both individual and group support. The appeal of this method for those who had experienced a loss led to a national network of support groups.

*Understanding the Dying Process* Several clinicians studied the dying trajectory, but it was Elisabeth Kübler-Ross whose name became a household word in connection with it. Her thesis on the psychological impact of impending death and her method of psychiatric intervention with dying patients became popular in the late 1960s. She advocated a warm, supportive approach to dying people, and she exposed the lonely, isolated way in which most people died. Her ideas served to encourage normalizing the dying process, but they also were interpreted as meaning that there was a healthy (acceptance of death) or pathological (denial of death) way to approach one's death. Kübler-Ross's research established a stage theory about the psychological process of dying. Some interpreted the theory as a directive for psychiatric interventions to assist people to work through their emotional responses to the dying process.

The first sign that her ideas had appeal came in 1965, when theological students at Billings Memorial Hospital asked her to offer a seminar about the psychological processes associated with death and dying. At that time, as a faculty member of the Chicago Medical School, she was interviewing dying patients. Her ideas were not well received by physicians, who frequently refused to allow her to work with their patients. But other members of the health care team were intrigued by her concepts of communication with dying people, and she was asked to share her ideas with these nonphysician health care professionals. Her reputation soon reached beyond the Chicago Medical School, and she was invited to lecture on her methods throughout United States. The publication of her book, *On Death and Dying,* in 1969 and an interview reported in *Life* magazine in 1970 enhanced the popularity of her ideas. Her ability to communicate the pathos of the dying person's situation aroused the public's sympathy, and she became the acclaimed spokesperson for the dying as well as a charismatic leader of the death with dignity and hospice movements in the United States.

Ed Schneidman also studied the psychological processes associated with death. He advocated a need for clinical thanatologists to help the average person deal with death—their own or the death of a loved one. He disagreed with Kübler-Ross's stage theory and suggested the following: "The dying person experiences a complicated clustering of intellectual and affective states, some fleeting, lasting for a moment, or a day, or a week, set not unexpectedly against the backdrop of that person's total personality, his 'philosophy of life' (whether an essential optimism and gratitude to life or a pervasive pessimism and dour or suspicious orientation to life)" (Schneidman 1973, 6). Suicide was Schneidman's special interest. He introduced the term "postvention" to describe the healing process necessary for survivors to overcome this traumatic loss.

*Recognizing the Special Needs of the Dying*  Providing special services for the terminally ill, which had begun in the mid-nineteenth century, reemerged during the 1950s and 1960s. Hospice care was only one response introduced at this time. This section examines some of the other approaches that were proposed to improve terminal care.

Dr. Jean Q. Benoliel, a nurse educator, researched and implemented a training method for clinical nurses called transition nursing, which emphasized continuity of care and open communication between patients and caregivers. The typical procedure in health care systems was to transfer patients back and forth from inpatient to outpatient services, depending on their needs, and nurses who provided their care changed depending on the setting. Benoliel recommended altering this practice; instead nurse practitioners were to maintain contact with their patients, regardless of health care setting. The nurse's role when working with a terminally ill patient was to follow the patient throughout the course of his or her illness and to help the patient understand what was occurring. Such consistency in care, Benoliel asserted, eased patients' anxiety and enabled them to work on understanding their illness. As they came to a better understanding they would be able to decide what treatment they wanted.

Dr. Melvin Krant directed another innovative program for terminally ill patients and their families—the Psychosocial Cancer Unit created at Tufts University in Boston in 1974. It was supported by a grant from the

National Cancer Institute "to study patterns of interaction between family, patient, and the larger society including the health care system, in the terminal phases of cancer, and to relate these patterns to bereavement outcomes in the years following death" (Krant, Beiser, Adler, and Johnson 1976, 116). Although developed as a research unit, professional staff also intervened to help patients and families prepare psychologically for death and to help families cope with their grief after death had occurred.

In India, Mother Teresa recognized the need for terminal care services. Her mission to aid India's poor included the establishment of 98 homes, and she created 60 more such facilities throughout the world. In Malaysia, Bishop Francis Chanlay, who was himself dying of cancer, raised funds to build the Mount Miriam Hospital for cancer patients. During his illness, Bishop Chanlay had received care from the Franciscan Sisters of Divine Motherhood, and he found their ministrations so soothing that before he died he wanted to ensure that others received similar care.

*Popularizing the Living Will*  In 1969 the Euthanasia Education Council, currently known as Concern for Dying, was formed by Charles Potter to disseminate information about the living will. By 1975 its membership had risen to 300,000, and 750,000 copies of the living will had been distributed (see figure 1). Consistent with many organizations in the death with dignity movement, which refrained from politicizing the problem, Concern for Dying's purpose is to educate, not legislate, the living will.

Public interest in living wills was sparked by the case of Karen Ann Quinlan, whose parents officially requested on 14 April 1975 that life support for their comatose daughter be withdrawn. Administrators at the facility that maintained Karen on a respirator were troubled by the request, and the case went to court. As a result of this case, questions such as "who determines treatment?" and "when should it cease?" became topics of widespread debate.

The living will allows the individual to decide, before becoming ill, in what circumstances he or she would not want aggressive treatment. California was one of the first states to initiate policies supporting patient control over treatment. The California Natural Death Act of 1976 permits the individual to refuse treatment. Since then more than 40 states have enacted statutes that recognize the living will.

Federal legislation enacted in 1991 supports the living will and the patient's right to determine treatment. The Patient Self-Determination Act,

---

**Figure 1   Living Will**

To My Family, My Physician, My Lawyer, and All Others Whom It May Concern:

Death is as much a reality as birth, growth, maturity, and old age—it is the one certainty of life. If the time comes when I can no longer take part in decisions for my own future, let this statement stand as an expression of my wishes and directions, while I am still of sound mind.

If at such a time the situation should arise in which there is no reasonable expectation of my recovery from extreme physical or mental disability, I direct that I be allowed to die and not be kept alive by mediations, artificial means, or "heroic measures." I do, however, ask that medication be mercifully administered to me to alleviate suffering even though this may shorten my remaining life.

This statement is made after careful consideration and is in accordance with my strong convictions and beliefs. I want the wishes and directions here expressed carried out to the extent permitted by law. Insofar as they are not legally enforceable, I hope that those to whom this Will is addressed will regard themselves as morally bound by these provisions.

**Durable Power of Attorney (optional)**

I hereby designate _____ attorney for the purpose of making medical treatment decisions. This power of attorney shall remain effective in the event that I become incompetent or otherwise unable to make such decisions for myself.

Signed _____
Optional notarization: Date _____
"Sworn and subscribed to Witness _____ before me this _____
day of _____, 1992," Witness _____
Notary public seal address _____
Copies of this request have been given to _____
(Optional) My Living Will is registered with Concern for Dying (No. _____).

---

Source: Concern for Dying.

---

sponsored by Sen. John Danforth, requires staff in hospitals and nursing homes to routinely ask patients how they want to spend their last days, and if they want to designate a health care proxy (a person to speak for the patient when he or she cannot). Although health care providers may still have the authority to perform aggressive life-saving procedures, particularly if they believe such treatments will result in longer life, the patient and family are now in a stronger legal position to prevent situations like Karen Quinlan's from taking months or years to be resolved. It is also recommended that individuals who want their wishes carried out find personal physicians who agree to honor the living will (Dunkin 1990).

*The IWG* Until the late 1960s the various activities described above were unrelated. Individuals might know of one another's interests, but there was no unifying or legitimating body that brought participants together. The development of the International Work Group on Death, Dying, and Bereavement was an organizational exception in this uncoordinated, multipurpose social movement. The use of the term *work group* in the organization's title meant what it said; when meetings were called, people came prepared to work on a particular issue. One might characterize the IWG as a mobile think tank; its members, all experts in thanatology, discussed the dying problem. They have always focused on intellectual debate rather than hands-on implementation.

The origins of the IWG are attributed to professionals who during the 1950s spread the word that cultural attitudes toward death had become problematic (Fryer 1982). Drs. John Hinton, Elisabeth Kübler-Ross, Collin Murray Parkes, and Cicely Saunders were among those identified as key figures. John Fryer, the IWG's first chair, designated research, death education, hospice care, and concern with death and dying as the organization's major emphasis. The IWG's mission statement is: "To conduct meetings of workers active in the field of death, dying, and bereavement of which the level of competence is sufficiently high so that the atmosphere is one of shared collegiality and in which there is not an 'audience.' We [the IWG] must encourage and promote what is known" (Fryer 1982, 2).

Initially, the group was loosely structured. Members got together when and where they could. Florence Wald, dean of the Yale University School of Nursing, was among the first to bring together Saunders, Kübler-Ross, and Parkes at her home in Connecticut to discuss the problems related to care of the dying in the United States. Symposiums by Robert Fulton in Minnesota in 1967 and Robert Kastenbaum in Detroit in 1969 also served to assemble experts in thanatology. In 1968 Ars Moriendi, a forerunner of the IWG was established. Until 1976, when the Ars Moriendi ceased to exist, the group conducted educational workshops on death and dying in the Philadelphia area.

The IWG met formally for the first time in 1974 at Columbia, Maryland, and it established the accoutrements of organizational structure as officers were elected, a membership list was created, and criteria for affiliation were established. Participation was selective, membership was by invitation only, and applicants had to be expert in thanatology. The IWG continued in this fashion until 1979, when the group incorporated in Pennsylvania. IWG conferences are now held every 18 months in locations across the world, including China, Norway, the United States, and Great Britain.

Like the death with dignity movement, the IWG has a history that has not been well documented. While explanations of its evolution are vague, its character has always been clear. IWG members are leaders, not followers. Their individual status as experts made the group prone to personality clashes. Sessions can turn into battles as individuals try to maintain control of their turf, each expert having a personal agenda to promote. Unifying members to pursue a single issue is not in keeping with the group's character. Throughout its history the IWG has functioned as a facilitator of ideas, not an implementer. Individual members have held positions of power and influence, but as a group they have not attempted to institute change. The group remains a specialized think tank that publishes ideas for others to develop in whatever ways are available to them. For example, the IWG has published standards on the psychiatric treatment of the dying patient but has not pursued ways to enforce these standards.

Although the atmosphere at IWG meetings can at times be unproductively competitive, the composition of the group also has advantages. Benoliel suggests that the creativity of the membership and the broad nature of their interests allowed them to move with the times (personal communication). As new social issues emerged this organization turned its attention to studying them. In recent years the increase in deaths at the hands of terrorists and the psychological impact of such events have been topics at IWG meetings.

Hospice proponents are among the IWG's participants. Henry Wald and William Lamers, who played important roles in developing the first hospice programs in the United States, were chairs of the IWG, and Saunders and Kübler-Ross have been participants. Advocates of hospice care, however, were not content with thinking and talking about hospice care, they wanted to find ways to implement and legitimate their ideas. The drive of hospice advocates to realize their ideas was exemplified by the way that their interests began to dominate IWG meetings. IWG members became disgruntled, stating that hospice concerns were taking over the meetings. Consequently, some hospice advocates created a separate organization to further their cause.

Because IWG members were interested in sharing knowledge, not in negotiating with external forces to implement ideas, the hospice concept could be maintained in its ideal form within the IWG's auspices. As the hospice movement's formal organizations moved far afield from its initial reformist goals, early hospice advocates turned to the IWG as a place to rekindle their initial fervor and reassert their ideals.

**Death with Dignity Today**   The assertion that "the death with dignity movement is still in its coalescent stage and not moving fast" (Hefferman and Maynard 1977) remains an accurate characterization. The death with dignity movement continues to appeal to some, but its ultimate goal, normal or "good death," is not easily achieved. Public attention to matters of health or dying continue to shift back and forth depending on what group captures the public interest. Groups such as the Foundation of Thanatology persist, but their popularity has waned. As time passed many who believed in this movement's ideals transferred their interest and enthusiasm to other social concerns. Leaders continue to assert their beliefs, but progress as evidenced by programs or policies has not been achieved.

The rise and fall of interest in this topic makes establishing policy difficult. Although help for the bereaved is more available and the concept of a living will better known and more widely applied, attempts to institutionalize goals have been sporadic. Beliefs that science can conquer illness and that only physicians should determine treatment continue to predominate in American culture. Few training courses exist for mental health professionals on treatment of dying patients or grieving survivors, and medical education continues to lack meaningful courses on death education (Butler 1979; Weeks 1989).

As the 1970s came to a close, the cultural emphasis on social needs and naturalistic practice became less popular; interest in thanatology continued, but it was relegated to specialty groups whose audiences were small and self-selected. During the 1980s the pendulum swung back toward material acquisition, individual responsibility, and scientific advancement. American interest turned from "preparing for death" to "fighting for life." The public was attracted to practices that helped them to improve health and fight illness. The growing popularity of Norman Cousins, Bernie Siegal, and Carl O. Simonton attests to changing social interests. Their writings encouraged individuals who suffered from serious illnesses to change their life-style and focus on the quality of life. Furthermore, they asserted that by directing one's psychic energy toward altering destructive attitudes, disease processes could be controlled. In keeping with cultural beliefs in the power of science, these prescriptions have been interpreted to mean that the individual can stave off disease or bring about remission when disease occurs.

As noted earlier, the concept of "good death" has reemerged in the 1990s. One reason is the increase in suicide among those who suffer from AIDS or Alzheimer's disease. The public expects to take part in decision-making processes, including the decision to take one's own life. Physicians, too, have begun to accept the value of discussing patients' wishes regarding aggressive treatments.

## A Hospice Movement Develops

Among the participants of the death with dignity movement were some who were particularly concerned with the treatment of terminally ill patients. Individuals working in the health care system observed that dying patients and their families did not receive the attention they needed. The discovery of various treatments, such as radiation therapy for cancer patients, resulted in people receiving treatments even though they had no hope of cure. As one leader of the hospice movement said, "Following World War II, the drive was to vanquish disease, as a result, the person who wasn't going to get well was lost sight of."

**The Influence of Cicely Saunders** It was within this context that Cicely Saunders introduced her comprehensive methods of terminal care. Saunders envisioned a method of care that employed physical, spiritual, and emotional support to improve the quality of life for dying patients and their families. In the 1940s, while employed as a social worker, Saunders met a Polish emigre, David Toma, who was dying. She saw him throughout the course of his illness, and they talked about what might ease the distress of dying. He bequeathed to her the sum of 50 pounds to be used for the purchase of a window in the facility for the terminally ill that they had imagined together. Following this experience Saunders resolved to become a physician and devote herself to the care of dying people.

Before entering medical school she volunteered at a hospice called Saint Luke's. While there she discovered that the sisters who attended dying patients had a unique way of administering medications; they gave them out around the clock instead of waiting until the patient was in pain. When Saunders became one of 20 research fellows studying methods of pain control, she used the knowledge gained at Saint Luke's to develop an analgesic research trial on pain management and symptom control.

On completing her medical degree Saunders became a medical officer at Saint Joseph's Hospice, where she implemented her philosophy of hospice care. Saunders believed that Western culture failed to acknowledge or comfort the dying. Caregivers must listen carefully to patients' complaints, she asserted, and explore ways to reduce them. Rather than treating symptoms and complaints with the expectation that little could be done to alleviate them, Saunders recommended careful attention to positioning, dietary preferences, and massage. Surgical techniques and radiation therapy were also used, not to cure disease but to relieve symptoms. Moreover, Saunders asserted that spiritual and emotional comfort were of equal importance in appropriate care of the dying.

In 1963 a grant from Saint Thomas's Hospice in London allowed Saunders to introduce her concept of hospice care to Americans. On this tour, Saunders visited 18 facilities and met people who were so impressed with her ideas and enthusiasm that they invited her to return repeatedly to assist them in spreading the word about hospice care. Before coming to the United States, Saunders contacted hospitals and parishes in this country to arrange a lecture tour, and in her letter she described her work, emphasizing her espousal of a comprehensive method of care that included spiritual care. This concern for spiritual care may have diminished physicians' interest in her work. Those who came to her lectures were primarily ministers, nurses, social workers, and other support staff.

To convert her audience to her cause, Saunders showed slides of patients before and after they received hospice treatments. The slides depicted patients who had been debilitated and disfigured by their symptoms transformed into people clearly capable of enjoying whatever time remained for them. According to Saunders, all cancer patients' pain and discomfort was treatable if properly diagnosed (Saunders 1981).

The visual portrayals of patients before and after hospice care were powerful. Saunders was acclaimed as "the angel come with a message" and as the "guiding star of the hospice movement" (Ogg 1985). Audiences found it hard to believe they were seeing cancer patients in the terminal stages of their illness. These patients appeared comfortable, alert, and able to interact with those around them—a far cry from what a patient undergoing aggressive radiation or chemotherapy looked like. Nonphysician health care workers who were troubled by the treatment of the terminally ill in hospitals saw hospice care as a possible solution. Some members of the death with dignity movement began to focus on the notion of hospice care as a way to achieve "death with dignity."

**Introducing a British Method to American Health Care**   One of the unanticipated problems the movement faced was that of integrating a British model of care into the American health care system. The movement's original leaders wanted to imitate Saunders's hospice, but that was not to be. The beliefs and values that influence American health care services are not the same as those in Great Britain. As we'll see in future chapters, in the United States the physical components of hospice care would overshadow emotional and spiritual support. Before continuing with the history of the hospice movement's emergence, let us briefly examine the differences between these two countries and the way that these differences affected the movement's evolution in the United States.

The modern concept of hospice care advocated by Saunders was consistent with British attitudes regarding acceptance of death and service to others. The American practice of using life-prolonging measures even when death is inevitable is as incomprehensible to the British as their pragmatic approach to death is to us (Falk 1984). The attendees at Saunders's lectures liked what she had to say, but they did not appreciate the effect philosophical differences might have on implementing hospice programs in America. They assumed that hospice ideals, because they were "right," would be approved by the American public and that physicians would therefore be forced to adopt hospice care.

The British are accepting of health care policies that restrict access to aggressive treatments, whereas Americans are not (Smith and Granbois 1982). For example, British patients over the age of 45 typically do not receive renal dialysis because the National Health Service has limited funds to support this service. In America people who suffer end-stage renal disease are able to receive Medicare benefits that support long-term dialysis treatments, regardless of their age or prognosis.

What Saunders labeled appropriate care U.S. physicians saw as an absence of treatment. As Saint Christopher's Hospice in London there were no temperature, pulse, and blood pressure rounds. No IVs were given, no blood samples taken (Holden 1978).

There are times when the treatment for a haemorrhage is not a blood transfusion with its attendant alarms but instead an injection and someone who stays there. There are infusions which should never have been put up; feelings of thirst can be relieved by the right use of narcotics. It is far better to have a cup of tea given slowly on your last afternoon than to have drips and tubes in all directions. This is not ineffectual sentimentality but proper care with all the compassionate matter-of-factness that the nuns at Saint Joseph's Hospice and many other experienced nurses have shown us over the years. (Saunders 1976, 3)

In the United States, technology rules health care. Giving out medications, conducting rounds, and drawing blood samples are important functions. Where technology is less necessary, such as in nursing homes, providers maintain the routines and norms of the acute health care system as if on constant guard, waiting for illness to occur.

British physicians are also different from American physicians in terms of their status and the nature of their interactions with patients. Saunders presented a comprehensive approach to the care of the dying (physical, spiritual, and emotional) that as a British physician she was willing to carry out, not write as an order for ancillary staff.

One explanation for the two countries' attitudinal differences toward death is that unlike Americans, the British witnessed death at home during two world wars. Limited exposure to natural disaster and increased life expectancy has fostered a belief among Americans that technology can overcome everything, including death (Smith and Granbois 1982).

The differences in attitudes toward technology were not the only aspects of hospice care that were inconsistent with American health care. The value of spirituality and the importance of volunteers conveyed by Saunders also were atypical of American health care. Although those who heard Saunders were impressed by her spirituality, it was not something they could simply implement in a program. Therefore, depending on who sponsored a program and where it developed, providers might or might not accept the importance of spirituality. The notion of using volunteers in a professional capacity was also uncommon in the United States. For the British, giving service is part of a tradition of noblesse oblige. Americans generally place more importance on work roles; volunteers have lower status and their activities are restricted. In England, having volunteers provide direct services is an accepted practice. In America, volunteers are more likely to stuff envelopes or conduct bake sales; they are rarely allowed to provide direct services (Osterweis and Champagne 1979).

Finally, British providers of hospice care were opposed to integrating with the acute health care system. They believed the National Health Service would exploit a terminal care unit, and during the 1960s and 1970s they kept hospice care separate from hospital care.

I do not see a special terminal ward within a general hospital as a good solution, either. Those nurses who did not want to do this kind of work would dread being posted to the ward and would not be the right people to work in it. Matron (or do I mean chief, principal, or senior nursing officer?) would be overheard to say 'I can't help it, we have three nurses off sick in the acute surgical ward: they'll have to be brought from the Dead End.' Consequently the terminal unit would be permanently understaffed. (Lamerton 1975, 156)

As programs proliferated the differences between British and American values and attitudes became obvious, particularly as programs became integrated with traditional health care systems.

**The Hospice Prototype**  Saint Christopher's Hospice opened in Syndenham, England, in 1967. In this first modern hospice, Saunders combined many features of traditional hospices with her innovative treatments for the terminally ill. The result was a facility designed to ensure one's comfort in a homelike environment.

To the arriving volunteer, it is a puzzle of major proportions at first to understand which is doctor, which is nurse, which is social worker, seminarian, psychiatrist, administrative assistant, steward, or secretary; and even in the wards themselves it is not always easy to be certain at first glance who is sick and who is well. Saint Christopher's is first and foremost a community; and it is a community of individuals. (Stoddard 1978, 70)

Instead of a terminal care or "death-house" environment with cachectic, narcoticized, bedridden, depressed patients, I found an active community of patients, staff, and families, and children of staff and patients. . . . Each bed has a colorful curtain around it, and there are some transparent, partial panels. Personal touches, such as flowers, paintings, comfortable lounge chairs, and wood, give a feeling of warmth. In addition to wards, there are family rooms for visits and a large room for group activities. (Liegner 1975, 1047)

The staff found that to put a patient in a window bed was one of the best cures for depression, along with providing a garden to which patients could be taken into the sunshine. In the garden there is a metal plaque in memory of the cancer patient who left his money to start the place, and playing in the garden—invited there as part of the therapy—one finds children of various races, cheering the patients with the sort of happy noise which is excluded from a hospital ward. (Rossman 1977, 85)

Professionals interested in developing hospice programs came to Saint Christopher's to observe its methods. In 1973 Saint Christopher's opened a study center, a separate building containing a library, bookshop, auditorium, and seminar rooms. Videos, training manuals, and lectures provided visitors with information about the use of technology for palliative care. In keeping with the communal environment of the hospice, visitors stayed at a nearby residence so they could absorb the atmosphere of the facility while learning its methods.

**The Influence of Elisabeth Kübler-Ross** Elisabeth Kübler-Ross's theory on the psychic stages a person passes through from the point of first learning he or she is terminally ill—consisting of denial, anger, bargaining, depression, and acceptance—is now well established in the psychiatric literature. In 1965 it was highly innovative. Kübler-Ross, a psychiatrist, asserted that as dying people experienced these different emotional stages they needed to communicate what they were feeling. Moreover, her experiences in hospital wards indicated that patients knew their prognosis and wanted to talk about it. Encouraging open discussion about dying, Kübler-Ross argued, enabled people to accept death and to face it peacefully.

In 1966 Saunders and Kübler-Ross were invited to lecture at Yale University Hospital by Florence Wald. They lectured separately, each presenting her own ideas about death and dying. Saunders emphasized the spiritual and physical aspects of care, Kübler-Ross the psychological. Kübler-Ross became interested in hospices as places where dying patients and families would have an environment conducive to talking about death. This interest led her to become a leader of the hospice movement in America.

Had Kübler-Ross not become involved in the movement, it might not have become as popular as it did. Saunders's concept of hospice care appealed to health care professionals, but Kübler-Ross made the public sit up and take notice of death and dying. Many were attracted to her ideas, regardless of whether they were interested in hospice care; her lecture tours are credited with inspiring the development of local seminars about death, dying, and grief.

Kübler-Ross's ideas were particularly attractive to the middle class. Theoretically, anyone could benefit from hospice care methods, but it was the educated, middle-class person who sought opportunities to talk about feelings and who sought services to improve quality of life. Studies about who received hospice services found that the typical patient was a middle-class, well-educated woman in her mid-50s suffering from breast cancer (Buckingham and Lupu 1982).

Kübler-Ross's influence and her belief in hospice care were such that she was able to convert other key figures to her views. William Lamers, a psychiatrist and founder of the Marin County hospice program in California, is a good example of this recruitment process. Lamers, through a personal experience with grief, wanted to improve psychological assistance for survivors. Like others in the death with dignity movement, Lamers felt that our culture did not appreciate people's need to process grief. To compensate for this cultural limitation, he conceived of a Center for Reaction to Loss (Stoddard 1978). While lecturing about grief reactions he met Kübler-Ross, who convinced him that hospice care would be a better way to accomplish his goals. Following her suggestion, he founded Hospice of Marin, one of the first hospice programs in this country.

**Spreading the Word about Hospice Care**   As Elisabeth Kübler-Ross and Cicely Saunders continued to lecture and attract a following, supporters organized into groups. Meetings held in churches, hospitals, and universities were common in the 1960s. The purpose of these meetings was not just to educate but to encourage an emotional attachment to the cause and to help those working with the dying cope with the stress of watching patients die, often in great discomfort, because of the nature of their disease or the medical treatment prescribed.

A typical meeting included slides or movies depicting patients who had been assisted to communicate about their death or had received pain management and symptom control techniques. Next, small group discussion encouraged participants to elaborate on the ideas generated by the visual presentation. Attendees shared their experiences of caring for terminally ill patients, and toward the end of the day they gathered in a large common room for tea and coffee and discussed their reactions to the meeting. Sometimes a few guitar players encouraged people to sing popular folk tunes, thus bonding the audience together in a shared emotional experience and recruiting members to the movement.

The audience such meetings attracted was selective. Ministers, nurses, psychiatrists, social workers, and those who had suffered the loss of a loved one made up the bulk of the attendees. Physicians and those suffering from chronic or terminal illness were not present.

## The Central Conflict of the Hospice Movement

As noted previously, the social conditions that encouraged the hospice movement's rise were multidimensional; they also were contradictory. As the hospice movement became a social cause separate from the death with dignity movement, its ideology was also formed. Combining interests in normalizing death with new treatments to ease its discomforts brought together two significant, albeit contradictory, perspectives; medicalizing and demedicalizing. The following paragraphs explore the importance of ideology and the way that it affected the hospice movement.

The part that grievance, or ideology, plays in a movement's accomplishments is much debated among social movement theorists. Mauss (1975) and resource mobilization theorists (McCarthy and Zald 1973) assert that social problems are constants and that belief systems are insufficient to bring about collective action. Although traditional social movement theory assumes that "shared grievances and homogenizing ideologies are important preconditions for the emergence of a social movement, resource mobilization theorists reject what they regard as the traditionalists' excessively psychological perspective" (Walsh 1981, 1–2).

New social movement theorists (Klandermans, Kriesi, and Tarrow 1988) have reasserted the importance of grievance, or ideology, to the rise of social movements, but they fail to analyze the way such ideas influence a social movement's course. "Ideational elements tend to be treated in primarily descriptive rather than analytical terms" (Snow and Benford 1988, 197). To treat the ideology, the values or beliefs, of the hospice movement descriptively would be to ignore a key factor affecting participation and the implementation of the movement's goals.

The beliefs that supported the emergence of the hospice movement were derived from both medicalizing and demedicalizing perspectives. Medicalization is said to occur when one labels behaviors or conditions as illnesses and then establishes treatments or cures performed in special environments by trained experts. Demedicalization results in the rejection of illness labels and treatments, and behaviors or conditions are attributed to moral failings or natural events. The hospice movement ideology was a composite of assertions that death's pains could be treated and cured, giving professionals control over the process (a medicalized perspective), and that death had to be normalized, returning control of the process to dying patients and their families (a demedicalized perspective).

Typically, a movement's mission is to right the social injustice that participants believe exists, and movement leaders take an extreme position against whatever condition in society they seek to influence, even though they may be willing to accept a moderated version of change. For example, prolife activists insist that abortion is wrong in any form and that all abortions must be forbidden. Some participants in the movement will actually agree with such an extreme position, but many prolife advocates would accept that abortion is permissible under certain conditions, particularly when there is a danger to the mother's health or when the pregnancy occurs as the result of rape. (A failed attempt in spring 1991 by the Utah legislature to ban abortion and prosecute women who sought abortions exemplifies this theory. Although the legislature asserted that abortion should be illegal, it took exception in cases of rape, incest, and danger to the mother's life.)

The mission of the hospice movement was to reform medical care by creating an alternative environment for dying patients. In the United States the movement took an idiosyncratic twist as it sought to return control of the dying process to the patient and family while it concomitantly attempted to introduce pain control techniques into medical practice. The movement's leaders never took a firm stand against hospitals, and therefore they did not encourage patients and families to reject acute health care services. To the contrary, some movement leaders integrated programs within the acute health care system.

Integrating these two perspectives created a paradox within the movement; proponents of hospice care advocated patients' right to die naturally while also advocating the use of biological and psychological techniques to treat them. The point here is not to establish whether the dying process was humanized or pain eased, it is to demonstrate how the integration of the two perspectives compromised the movement's ideals. The contradictions inherent in a belief system that incorporates medicalizing and demedicalizing viewpoints inhibited participants' ability to collectively take a side for or against acute health care practices.

From the earliest stages of the movement, hospice leaders were unclear. Did hospice philosophy favor or oppose the acute health care system? This lack of resolve blurred the movement's mission and attracted a diverse group of supporters. This in turn made the movement vulnerable to external forces and affected the implementation of hospice programs. Some programs medicalized dying, others demedicalized it, but it was difficult to do both.

A movement's ideology also affects participation. New social movement theorists assert that social movement participants and their beliefs have changed. Socially displaced malcontents seeking to revolutionize society do not make up the constituency of contemporary movements; rather, a new middle class concerned about the negative consequences of modernity have become participants in contemporary movements. The nature of the international hospice movement's ideology and participants is consistent with new social movement theory. As increased life span and its companion, chronic debilitating illness, became commonplace in Western civilization, an affluent middle class sought ways to provide humane care for victims of these conditions.

Those attracted to the American hospice movement contributed to its ambiguity of purpose. For the most part hospice leaders emerged from within hospital environments, where they had been socialized to value medical science. Therefore, many hospice leaders were ambivalent; should dying patients be freed from hospital environments, or could medical science ease their discomfort? Consequently, movement participants did not assemble for protest marches, and leaders did not make speeches asserting the dangers of medical science; the movement could hardly attack a system it embraced.

Contradictory forces within the movement facilitated its rise, but altered its accomplishments. Ultimately, most American hospice programs had as much in common with traditional health care services as they did with their original philosophy. Politically the movement favored integrating hospice programs with hospitals because this strategy enabled providers to gain access to health care dollars. But existing in a medical environment meant downplaying or even ignoring other aspects of hospice care, such as bereavement and spiritual services. As integration with mainstream medicine began to dominate the movement, those programs that did not integrate had difficulty surviving, and so there were fewer such programs.

The hospice movement flourished in a social environment that encouraged medicalizing and demedicalizing perspectives, and an appreciation for the movement's dilemma is rooted in the nature of these perspectives. Although usually in opposition, these two viewpoints are not always mutually exclusive, as can be seen from the hospice movement's experience. Medicalizing and demedicalizing trends coexist, and there is considerable ambivalence toward them in the United States. As categories of illness broaden, societal balances regarding who is responsible and who is in control changes (Fox 1979; Sedgwick 1982).

The coexistence of strong medicalizing and demedicalizing trends suggests that considerable ambivalence exists in the United States about how broadening the categories of illness and the sick role is affecting societal balances between exemptions and controls and rights and responsibilities. A striking legal expression of this ambivalence can be found in the "guilty, but mentally ill" verdict that a series of states have added to their statutes during the 1980s. In effect, the concept of "guilty, but mentally ill" attempts to combine criminal culpability with sick role exemptions. (Fox 1989, 30)

The following sections describe medicalizing and demedicalizing trends to further clarify this ideological dilemma.

**Medicalization**   As noted earlier, medicalization is said to occur when behaviors or social phenomena are defined as illness and medical treatments are established to cure them. Medicalizing processes are not a consequence of health care needs; rather, they serve to change our perception from "badness" to "sickness." As the definitions of illness and health have expanded, "conviction has grown that health and health care are rights rather than privileges, signs of grace, or lucky, chance happenings. In turn, these developments are connected with higher expectations on the part of the public about what medicine ideally ought to be able to accomplish and to prevent" (Fox 1979, 467). Consequently, "all kinds of problems now roll up at the physician's door, from sagging anatomies to suicides, from unwanted childlessness to unwanted pregnancy, from marital difficulties to learning difficulties" (Kass 1975, 11). Criminality becomes a conduct disorder, drunkenness becomes alcoholism, and overactivity in childhood becomes hyperkinesis.

Associating such conditions with health care lends them the aura of importance that surrounds medical practice in this country. "Medical treatments for deviant behavior are heralded frequently as examples of the 'progress' typical of modern society, believed to unfold in a linear fashion, leaving beneficial advances in its wake" (Conrad and Schneider 1980, 33). Furthermore, being considered sick rather than lazy or evil absolves one of responsibility for one's circumstances. A disease is a condition over which one has no control; to be cured, one must turn oneself over to the medical experts.

The profitable industry created by a society that seeks to cure diseases further contributes to, and reaps the benefits of, medicalization (Conrad and Schneider 1980), thus reinforcing the need to maintain this construction of reality. Believing that behaviors such as drinking, hyperactivity, and antisocial behavior are diseases and crediting medical science with the ability to cure them has created a treatment industry that holds onto its market share tightly.

Concomitant with, and partially responsible for, the expanding definition of disease has been the rise of physicians as determiners and controllers of illness labels and treatments (Freidson 1970a). Physicians, through a series of political strategies, improved their status by redefining physical processes such as birth and aging as medical events, and they eliminated competition from other health care providers such as midwives or barber surgeons by claiming that only university-trained physicians should intervene in matters of health (Starr 1982). "The medical profession has first claim to jurisdiction over the label illness and anything to which it may be attached, irrespective of its capacity to deal with it effectively" (Freidson 1970b, 251).

Physician dominance alone, however, does not explain the medicalization of American culture; consumer demand and belief in these treatments has also played a part. As Zola stated, "for if none of these [i.e., the list of activities or behaviors labeled health or illness] obtained today we should still find medicine exerting an enormous influence on society. The most powerful empirical stimulus for this is the realization of how much everyone has or believes he has something organically wrong with him, or put more positively, how much can be done to make one feel, look, or function better" (1978, 258). Fox referred to this as "the assumed right of members of society to 'health,' 'quality of life,' and 'quality of death' " (1979, 473).

**Demedicalization**     By the 1960s a countertrend, demedicalization, had developed. This countertrend was a response to what was felt to be a state of "overmedicalization" (Fox 1979). Disease labels had consequences for the individuals so labeled. Although sick people are expected to put themselves under professional control and are not held responsible for their condition, this legitimizing of their illness has its price: they are expected to recover as expeditiously as possible (Parsons 1972, 108).

This recognition that disease labels had negative consequences resulted in attempts to remove the stigmatizing and dehumanizing affects of such labels.

Uneasiness about the "power" and "control" exercised by a "dominant" medical profession, concern about the way in which applying the concept of illness and therapy to an ever-widening gamut of attitudes and behaviors may be eroding the "right to be different," and criticism of the powerlessness, ostracism, dehumanization, and even "mortification of the self" that the label sick may imply, have been persistently voiced. (Fox 1989, 29)

Advocates of demedicalization emphasized normalizing conditions labeled diseases; the recategorizing of homosexuality from a form of mental illness to an alternative life-style is one example of this trend. A surge in consumer demand for alternative services such as home birthing, holistic medicine, and self-help services in the 1960s and 1970s also represented attempts to regain control over health and live a "normal life" (Conrad and Schneider 1980). Improving community and family supports, it was claimed, could do more to reduce the incidence of alcoholism and antisocial behavior than medical treatment (Peele 1989).

Demanding accountability for physician practice was a secondary consequence of demedicalization; consumers expected the medical profession to be more carefully scrutinized and recipients of health services to have access to information about treatments.

According to those espousing this view, categorizing conditions as diseases and subsequently treating them became an overused and expensive practice in America that did little to improve health. Most diseases are self-limiting, and treatments often succeed because of a placebo effect (Illich 1976; Peele 1989). Illich stated that medical science has created as many diseases as it supposedly has cured, and people would do better to take more responsibility for their well-being. He concluded, "hospital 'worship' is unrelated to the hospital's performance" (1976, 106).

**An Unresolved Paradox**  From its earliest stages the movement's conflicting beliefs fostered an internal co-optation process. Leaders were influenced by medicalizing ideas, demedicalizing ideas, or both, and they unwittingly attempted to merge these concepts in hospice programs.

The hospice movement's ideology emphasized "good death," one free from the array of technological interventions that had become part of standard operating procedures in the care of the dying. Thus, hospice advocates encouraged demedicalizing and deprofessionalizing the dying process. Yet hospice advocates also believed technology could ease pain and discomfort. Although hospice leaders agreed that medical treatments were overused and that patients died in isolation and discomfort because they were treated as if curable up to the last minutes of their lives, it was difficult for them to stand firm against the health care system; they also believed that medical technology could benefit patients by reducing their physical pain, and they wanted American physicians to accept this application of medical technology. Thus, hospice advocates fostered the addition of new technologies that medicalized and professionalized the treatment of the dying.

By medicalizing hospice programs, leaders made them attractive to health care providers and consumers for reasons other than the movement's original intent. Ascribing treatments to dying patients and families made hospice care the domain of physicians, although movement participants simultaneously asserted that physicians were incapable of properly caring for dying patients. Integrating hospice care with hospitals as an expedient way to create programs attracted the attention of medical entrepreneurs, but they were interested in hospice programs as a way to expand the health care industry. Furthermore, a culture that deified science and increasingly clamored for more treatments to ease every social, psychological, and physical symptom it experienced was also interested in hospice care. Better educated patients and families who became aware of hospice treatments requested such services to ease their physical and psychological pain.

The ambivalence that our society experiences toward medicalizing and demedicalizing processes also affected the hospice movement. Although hospice leaders avowed that the American public was ready for reform of terminal care, this point of view was more a wish than a reality. As Freidson (1985) pointed out, debates about controlling physician practice that appear in the literature still reflect writers' desire to deprofessionalize medical practice rather than an actual trend. Therefore, leaders of the hospice movement who misconstrued the demand for change as being indicative of actual reforms would be disappointed by the public's response. The public did not clamor for hospice services; rather, a minority constituency perceived that such a service was desirable.

Ultimately, hospice providers achieved only a few of their stated goals. One of their unanticipated but major accomplishments was to expand the health care industry. Medicalizing forces dominated hospice care in ways that its advocates had not foreseen, and most programs became little more than extensions of the health care industry. Demedicalizing processes, such as assisting dying AIDS patients or improving worker satisfaction, succeeded insofar as they did not affect medical treatments. Controversial practices, such as encouraging patients, families, and caregivers to acknowledge and talk about death, were carried on covertly by some participants but were not part of the movement's political agenda.

Early participants in the movement were seeking validation of their concerns for the plight of the dying, and they did not anticipate future conflicts. Nor did they oppose one another's ideas as these conflicts arose—rebels who wanted to reform the health care system joined with health care professionals who supported the introduction of new treatments. Individuals enjoyed a supportive atmosphere where they could discuss concerns about which they had been silent, and their sense of mission made them tolerant of all who shared their desire to improve conditions for the dying. Lack of appreciation for the contradictory nature of the movement's philosophy facilitated its progress toward the next stage of its development, coalescence. Had individuals stopped to examine their ideology, they might not have forged ahead in the way that they did to implement programs in whatever setting would have them.

## Conclusion

Initially, hospice care was one social movement organization within the death with dignity movement. During the late 1960s hospice proponents separated their cause from the death with dignity movement, and a core membership developed whose purpose was to institutionalize hospice care in the United States. The charisma of Cicely Saunders and Elisabeth Kübler-Ross inspired their followers with emotional zeal and mobilized them to want to improve conditions for terminally ill patients and their families.

From the outset the movement was beset by two difficulties that were to stay with it. First, the American movement borrowed heavily from Saunders's ideas about hospice care, which were far more compatible with the values and attitudes toward health care held by the British than by Americans. Second, and perhaps most important, the hospice movement's mission was essentially paradoxical: to humanize care for the dying and their families *and* to introduce new forms of medical technology to ease the pain of death.

Thus, from its inception, the hospice movement contained the seeds of its future failings. In this movement the co-optive forces that are usually initiated by external forces came from within. The movement essentially co-opted itself. The attempt to introduce a British concept of care, the lack of a clear values statement, and the differing beliefs of core members resulted in a blurring of the movement's mission as leaders attempted to implement their ideas.

*Chapter 5*

# Creating the First Modern Hospice Programs

The opening of the first modern hospice, Saint Christopher's, in Sydenham, England, in 1967 inspired clergy and health care workers in the United States such as Florence Wald, Carlton Sweetser, and William Lamers to assemble groups to talk about hospice care and the psychology of death and dying. These meetings resulted in the creation of the first modern American hospice programs. Concurrently, a national assembly of hospice supporters created the first political organization of the hospice movement, the Hospice National Advisory Council. These activities are consistent with the coalescent phase of a social movement; leaders emerge, participants are recruited, and organizations are created to implement ideals. Then, as the activities of the organizations are publicized, the public becomes aware that a new social problem exists. The end of the hospice movement's coalescent stage was marked by the start of the first three hospice programs.

## Participation in the Hospice Movement

During its coalescence the ideology of a social movement is translated into some form of action, certain individuals are identified as leaders, and their promotion of the cause convinces other members of society to participate. Mauss (1975) defines three levels of participation in a social movement; the leaders, the active membership, and the benefactors.

The leaders are those participants most committed to the movement's goals, and as the movement progresses they are often viewed as zealots or fanatics. Elisabeth Kübler-Ross and Cicely Saunders were the charismatic leaders of the hospice movement; others, such as Florence Wald, Edward Dobihal, William Lamers, and Carlton Sweetser, actually developed the first programs in the United States. As the movement gained popularity, new leaders, such as Donald Gaetz and Dennis Rezendes, contributed to program proliferation, but they also accommodated policymakers' demands that hospice care be cost-effective.

The active membership are those participants who carry out the movement's goals but don't control its political process. Moreover, although they support the movement's mission, they may have secondary interests and may therefore be willing to accept deviations from the original ideals. Ministers, nurses, and those who had lost a loved one from cancer were the majority of participants in the hospice movement.

The benefactors are those participants who take up a movement while it is fashionable and then withdraw their support as they perceive that it has achieved its goals. These participants are most available during a social movement's incipience. The hospice movement's benefactors were the survivors of cancer patients and advocates of death with dignity who believed hospices would help as a way to bring death and dying out of the closet. The Hospice National Advisory Council and the International Work Group on Death, Dying, and Bereavement are other examples of the supportive benefactor. As hospice programs gained ground and the National Hospice Organization (NHO) formed, these participants withdrew from the movement's political process.

A social cause does not emerge and then simply attract people to it; rather, participants become interested in a social issue, and as they form groups to discuss it they also shape the definition of the problem and the strategies aimed at resolving it. Therefore, the identity and interests of the participants are important components of the analysis of a social movement's history. The constituents of the hospice movement had little power to bring about the reforms they sought, and they would not be the primary beneficiaries of these reforms. Let's now take a closer look at the participants—and some of the significant nonparticipants—in the hospice movement.

**Key Participants**  Clergy were at the forefront of concerned professionals who wanted change. Although grief was beginning to become an important topic psychologically, it was a long-standing concern of pastoral care. The clergy's presence in hospitals and their role in the dying process made them more in tune with what was occurring; they had ministered to dying patients and their families, and they were familiar with traditional hospices.

Saunders's reassertion of the concept of hospice care gave the clergy an acceptable way to improve treatment of the dying, but they lacked the power to enforce their ideas. Their role is to comfort the sick or dying and to pray with mourners; they are rarely asked to participate in decisions about treatment. (The exception is the unusual situation in which there is a moral or ethical concern, such as withdrawing life-support systems. Clergy do participate in discussing the issue, but the authority to make the decision still largely rests with the physician. See chapter 4 for a discussion of the legal issues attending withdrawal of life support.) The introduction of hospice programs could thus not be accomplished solely through the efforts of the clergy.

Nurses were also integral to program development in this country. Like the clergy, nurses traditionally have held supportive roles in the patient care process. But they, too, lacked the authority to implement their ideas. The hospice movement was not a women's movement per se, but there was perhaps an unspoken goal of empowerment for women—particularly nurses. Once established, hospice programs did serve as conduits for nurses' professional advancement. When hospice care became popular in the United States, nurses were just beginning to develop ways to improve their professional status (Greer and Mor 1985). Examples are the upgrading of nurses' education through B.S.N. and M.S.N. degree programs and their placement in positions outside the confines of acute care hospitals, where they took orders from physicians. Nurses had assumed leadership roles in other areas of health care, such as nursing homes, birthing clinics, and home health care agencies. Hospice programs, with their emphasis on supportive care, provided another avenue for advancement. The potential of hospice programs to give nurses more autonomy was facilitated by physicians' lack of interest in the programs.

Psychiatrists were also interested in this new concept of care, but they did not involve themselves in the politics of the movement. Hospices merely provided a place where they could implement their theories about psychiatric intervention with dying patients. Psychologists, though they were interested in thanatology, were unlikely team members. They were not a part of the traditional health care team, and, like psychiatrists, were more interested in treating emotional problems than in advancing social causes.

Another professional group interested in Saunders's ideas were social workers, who, like nurses and pastoral caregivers, had traditionally helped patients and families cope with terminal illness. They were interested in developing more humane treatments, particularly ones that acknowledged families' needs, but as a professional group they had little impact on the political process of the movement. As members of a conservative, institutionally based profession, social workers are rarely at the forefront of social movements. The move toward private practice since the 1970s has not increased the power of social workers to effect social reforms.

Finally, there were the families and friends of those who had died. Since death knows no boundaries of class or status, all social classes were represented in this group; some were influential people who were able to do more than just talk about hospice care. Members of this group were active in setting up hospice programs during the 1970s. They were part of the volunteer staff, and in the early days often the only staff. Although providing services for others may have helped members of this group complete their own mourning, it also improved conditions for others experiencing the stress associated with loss. Furthermore, it was from within this group that money was raised and political connections made.

For the most part, physicians were not among the movement's participants. Although physicians were often asked and agreed to serve on hospice boards, they were not among the early audiences who attended lectures about this concept of care. Physicians were not particularly interested in meeting the emotional or spiritual needs of the dying; that role had been the business of ancillary staff, nurses, pastoral counselors, and social workers. Physicians were more concerned that "the arbitrary designation of terminality might interfere with modern treatment techniques" (Schnaper and Wiernick 1983, 104).

Dying patients, the inspiration for Saunders's and Kübler-Ross's ideas about terminal care, were also missing from the roster of participants. The terminally ill were recipients of services, not agents of change. Their testimonies about the benefits of hospice care were used to advance the cause, but they did not take part in designing or implementing programs.

Their absence is also noticeable in the research on terminal care. Researchers during the past 20 years have studied dying people's feelings, but they typically ask the patient's family to respond for the patient (Wilkinson 1986). The absence of participation by those most concerned with the reform of this service, dying people, influenced the movement's achievements. Research on hospice care's accomplishments indicates that family stress is alleviated by this method, and, as stated earlier, families were in fact active participants in the hospice movement. These same studies did not report a similar outcome for patients.

**Key Leaders** Cicely Saunders and Elisabeth Kübler-Ross galvanized early support for the hospice movement. Yet while each is considered a charismatic leader, each played a different role. Fox described Kübler-Ross "as the advertent and Saunders as an inadvertent" charismatic leader of the American hospice movement (1980, ix), but these roles reversed as programs were implemented. Although Kübler-Ross made *hospice* a household word in this country, she did not take an active role in program planning and implementation. Saunders did offer hands-on assistance in organizing programs in America. The activities of these two women is exemplified by the following interview with a hospice program employee:

> "Dr. Saunders was wonderful. She came here and taught us how to set up charts, you know there were no manuals at that time. She spent a few days and talked to the staff about this [hospice] work."
>
> "Did Dr. Kübler-Ross also visit the program?"
>
> "Oh yes . . . I think so. Yes, she came once to give an in-service on death and dying, but Dr. Saunders was the one who really helped us."

Other participants concur with this account. While Saunders visited programs regularly and kept abreast of their progress, Kübler-Ross provided in-service education about communication with dying patients. Saunders's willingness to participate in resolving providers' pragmatic questions gave her greater influence over program design. She envisioned hospice care as credible medical care, and in America this concept was often translated to mean an emphasis on the management of physical symptoms rather than a multidimensional approach to physical, spiritual, and emotional distress.

While Saunders and Kübler-Ross were the charismatic leaders of the hospice movement, Florence Wald was its organizer. Zelda Foster, a member of the International Work Group on Death, Dying, and Grief, reported, "Florence was wonderful. She brought together those of us who had been working with dying people in hospital settings and who were feeling isolated and alone, and unable to do anything to improve the situation [for the terminally ill]" (personal communication).

Wald developed the Yale Study Group, and after succeeding with it she proceeded to contact people around the country who were interested in terminal care to see if they would like to participate in a group whose goal was to develop modern hospice programs nationally. After years of informal communication the group assembled in 1974 at the IWG's first official meeting in Baltimore. Among the members of this group were those who developed the first three hospice programs in the United States.

## Ambiguity of Purpose and Unsupported Claims: Consequences for the Movement

Ambiguity of purpose is the factor that helps us understand the choices core members made as they attempted to implement their ideas. The hospice movement was not a single-issue movement; its values conflicted and its participants had mixed allegiances. Normalizing death meant taking dying people away from medical settings where machines and drugs were used to prevent death; treating physical and emotional pain meant bringing people into the medical system where they could be assessed and treated.

Initially, hospice leaders wanted to imitate Saunders's facility, but funding was difficult to obtain. Core members' eagerness to start hospices encouraged them to explore alternatives. To accomplish their goal, program creation, they altered program form, so that not one but three program types were created. The first program began as a home care service, but eventually replicated the Saint Christopher's model. The second program was a team of health care professionals who oversaw dying patients' care in the hospital. The third, comprised chiefly of volunteer staff, provided supportive care for dying people in their homes. Adaptations in form changed the definition of hospice from a place of care to a concept of care that could be provided anywhere. These innovations were intended to be temporary, to get the movement off the ground, so to speak. Instead, these alternative forms were institutionalized.

Confounding the decision to participate in the acute health care system was the vision of the movement's leaders. Hospice care, as they perceived it, was a first step in revolutionizing the health care system; "hospice, with its emphasis on a multidisciplinary team of caregivers, challenges us to rethink our definition of medical care" (Silver 1980, 180). Someday palliative care practices would be incorporated into mainstream medical practice. "Of course one could hope that some day care of the dying will be so good, and so thoroughly taught to students, that hospices become obsolete because hospitals and family doctors cope without trouble" (Lamerton 1975, 156).

It is rare for a social movement to maintain purity of purpose. To propel the movement forward and implement their ideas, leaders find it necessary to compromise with political organizations outside their sphere of influence. Most providers believed they were achieving a victory by being able to integrate with an acute health care setting; hospice care could be provided anywhere. Some leaders recognized that there were problems associated with this integration, but the movement's political thrust, to create programs, overshadowed their concerns.

**Leaders Choose Diverse Paths** Lack of a clear purpose or a single issue on which the movement's leaders held firm resulted in different program developers inadvertently taking different positions vis-à-vis the acute health care system and emphasizing different aspects of hospice care. Although it was not the core members' intent, once they established treatments for the dying and integrated them with the acute health care system, that system became attractive to hospice care advocates for reasons that were not in keeping with the ideals of the movement. The needs of mainstream medicine dominated and subsumed hospice advocates' reform efforts.

Concomitantly, the humanistic, demedicalizing components of the movement's mission led to the development of programs that did not emphasize medical treatments for dying patients. Many who heard the lectures of Kübler-Ross were touched by the pathos of the dying person's plight, and they wanted to return death to a natural environment, the family home. Therefore, volunteers who might or might not have medical training set up community programs that offered supportive services. Their clientele was self selected; services were restricted to those in the community who had heard of the concept, wanted to die at home, and had a medical course that was uncomplicated.

**Advocating Hospice Care's Benefits** During the coalescent stage a movement's major task is to acquire resources in the form of a popular following, financial backing, and support from larger bureaucracies. One way that leaders acquire resources is by making claims regarding the need for reform. The veracity of their assertions, or leaders' ability to substantiate their claims, are not as important as one might think. Hospice supporters asserted the importance and popularity of their cause with little or no proof.

Hospice advocates stated that pain management could cure discomfort, despite that fact that there was little evidence to support such a claim (Holden 1978). Fear of pain and discomfort is the greatest fear people have about cancer (Hinton 1977), and therefore claims to alleviate them were appealing. Contradictory assertions that certain cancer illnesses were relatively free of pain and debilitation (Illich 1976) went unnoticed as the movement's leaders avowed that cancer patients died in pain and discomfort. This is not an attempt to prove or disprove whether cancer is accompanied by pain, but rather to point out the way that beliefs are constructed and then presented as facts.

Another assertion by core members was that the American public wanted hospice services. Again, little evidence supported this claim. The Yale Study Group conducted a community survey and reported that terminally ill people did not want aggressive, cure-at-all-costs treatments during the last days of their life. Furthermore, the group asserted that people preferred to spend their last days at home in familiar surroundings. The findings of this study were used to prove that hospice care was desired by the public; future researchers (Greer et al. 1986) were unable to replicate the results.

The following statements are examples of unsubstantiated claims made by hospice advocates. "Since the late 1960s a profound shift in attitudes toward dying and illness has occurred among consumers and providers of care for chronically ill. The hospice movement is gaining momentum in the United States as a reaction to the 'cure at any cost' medical treatment" (Carey 1986, 13–16). Others asserted that since 1974 hospice care had become popular in the United States; that hospice programs were alternatives to the acute health care system; or that since 1974 hospice programs had become a popular alternative to the acute care hospital for those suffering from terminal illness. One writer was even more affirmative: "Hospice will not become obsolete because those forces which create a need for it, high hospital costs, increasing health care mechanization, will continue to grow. More technological discovery in the fight against disease will only create a greater need for humanistic care" (Koff 1980, 5).

Statements by dying patients were also proffered as proof that hospice care was a desired alternative to the acute health care system.

In May 1973, Eugene C., a retired Navy warrant officer learned that he had cancer of the prostate. By last July, the pain had blossomed and was eating him alive. When the family doctor pronounced the illness terminal and suggested a nursing home, his wife reported "we couldn't stand seeing him suffer." At that point, many families would have given up and surrendered the patient to an institution, to die in a drugged stupor or in pain among strangers. Today, he strides about his own house free of pain and sharing fully in the life of his wife and sons for however long he has left. (Hospice, Inc., 1975, 1)

I know I am dying of cancer and am reconciled to this. I have come to a special hospital whose aim is the relief of pain among terminal and long-term patients. I know that nothing will be done to prolong life for me, only let death come as naturally and happily as possible. Since coming to the special hospital [Saint Christopher's], I have felt a new person, for when I was at the teaching hospital I really felt close to death and considered taking something to end it all. Here I have been able to do things I thought I would never do again. This has been the most enormous pleasure and I have enjoyed life once again. (Dunnet 1973)

These assertions attracted public attention and established the rightness of the movement's cause. They also gave its leaders a false sense of security; if society was so strongly in favor of hospice care, then the movement would have little difficulty succeeding in its intent.

## Early Organizations

**The First Planning Groups** Planning groups were common during this period, and they served to promote the concept of hospice care as well as to reinforce participants' belief in the importance of their mission. Wald and the Yale Study Group inspired the development of other local groups. There was a recurrent formula in the way these early community groups evolved. First, a member of a religious order, often an Episcopal priest, became interested in doing something about the dying problem. This person might be a hospital employee or a parish minister; his or her first step was to spread the word about hospice care. Community members and health care professionals were then recruited to form a hospice board.

Once the hospice board was assembled, its members met regularly to discuss the viability of creating a hospice program. This planning stage would usually last for 12 or 18 months. During that time the board would seek donations either to send members to England to learn more about Saunders's method of care or to hire someone to begin setting up a program. This person would not provide patient care, but would promote hospice concepts with hospital staff or members of the community and set up procedure manuals, service descriptions, and budgets. Following these initial activities the board would pursue other funding sources and obtain community sanctions to establish a hospice program. Once a program began providing patient care, board members turned their attention to maintaining funding or participating in national efforts to legitimize hospice programs.

Saint Christopher's Hospice in England became a mecca for those interested in hospice care. Florence Wald, Ed Dobihal, and several others from the Yale Study Group went to England to observe Saunders's methods. Others, such as hospital administrators whose support was needed to create programs, were sent to Saint Christopher's to convince them of the benefits of hospice care. A visit to the wards of Saint Christopher's was the best way to educate and convert skeptics. The sight of patients who had no hope of recovery but who appeared content was a powerful persuader.

One example of this conversion process was described by Rev. Sweetser of Saint Luke's Hospital in New York. Sweetser wanted to develop a hospice program at Saint Luke's, but he had trouble convincing the hospital's board of its value. In the early 1970s board member Bill Trent was planning a trip to England. Sweetser convinced him to visit Saint Christopher's and see for himself the importance of Saunders's work. Trent did so and, despite previous reservations, was impressed by what he observed. Upon his return to New York he contacted Sweetser and told him to begin plans to develop a hospice program at Saint Luke's.

Visitors to Saint Christopher's Hospice not only met Saunders, they found out about other groups that were attempting to develop hospice programs. For example, a minister from North Carolina who was interested in hospice care might go to Saint Christopher's to learn more about its program. While there he would learn of U.S. groups already implementing hospice programs that would be able to help him with the start-up process. These interactions strengthened the movement.

**The First Legitimizing Bodies** One measure of the movement's popularity and capacity for organization is evidenced by the creation of the Hospice National Advisory Council, its first political organization. The board met for the first time in 1974 and its chair was Elisabeth Kübler-Ross. Its membership comprised 124 community leaders, including physicians, politicians, thanatologists, and philanthropists. Its purpose was to establish the importance of hospice care and to support the creation of a nationwide network of hospice programs. "This council, composed of professionals and non-professionals with an interest in the health care delivery system in America, will provide national visibility for Hospice" (Hospice, Inc., 1974, 2).

As the concept of hospice care became popular another group, the National Hospice Organization, was created to promote the movement politically. The Hospice National Advisory Council persisted as an agent that brought together influential supporters, but it did not participate in establishing funding or regulating hospice programs.

## The Original Components of Hospice Care

Before describing the evolution of the first hospice program, let us examine the way that the hospice movement's leaders defined their ideals. They advocated a combination of medical treatments and naturalistic practices, making the hospice concept unlike other health care methods.

The modern hospice program was intended to address the emotional, physical, and spiritual needs of dying patients and their families. Modern hospices were not just comfortable places to spend one's last days but comprehensive treatment centers for terminally ill patients and their families. As groups created programs in America, they did not all give equal weight to each component of care. As the movement grew and programs proliferated there was a subversion of the ideals in some but not all the programs. The following sections describe the *original* components of the modern hospice program.

**Patient and Family as a Unit of Care**  A central theme of hospice philosophy was that the patient and family were the unit of care. Traditional medical care separated patient needs from family needs and focused attention on the physical aspects of disease. Hospice philosophy emphasized that dying was a life experience, not a medical event, and that people's emotional and spiritual needs were equally important. Furthermore, families, too, were affected by terminal illnesses, and family support was a component of care.

As Dr. Josefina Magno, past president of the National Hospice Organization, explained, "You find the families are full of unanswered questions.

Doctors, nurses simply don't have time to handle them. So they're left to wonder: Will their relatives smother to death, will there be much bleeding or pain or disfigurement?" (Cherry 1982, 313). Hospice staff members were trained to listen and respond to such questions.

Bereavement counseling was another way hospice teams met families' emotional needs. Grief work following a patient's death was part of the healing process, and hospice caregivers, because they were not part of a traditional health care team that ceased being involved once a patient had been cured or had died, continued their involvement with family and friends as long as they were needed.

The case of Mrs. S., who after 40 years of marriage had become a widow, exemplifies this component of hospice care. Prior to her husband's death, Mrs. S. had focused on his needs, and she had pushed aside the team's efforts to discuss her feelings and fears. The team knew that avoiding discussion about death frequently led to a stronger than usual grief reaction. They visited Mrs. S. the day after the funeral and explained to her that their services did not end with her husband's death, and she accepted their offer of assistance. Mrs. S. experienced the death of her husband as the loss of the best part of herself. She would often start an activity or a thought as if her husband was still alive, and then realize that he was not. Hospice workers encouraged Mrs. S. to speak freely about her husband, something that she was not encouraged to do by others. Furthermore, the team did not treat her behavior as a sign of mental illness. For a time, they helped fill the void left by her husband and allowed her to make the transition from spouse to widow.

**Patient Participation in Treatment** One way to counteract the physician-dominated, technologically oriented health care system and return control to the individual was to educate patients and give them choices about their treatment options. Patients were encouraged to decide where they wanted to spend their remaining days, and staff educated them about the different medical procedures that could be used to treat their symptoms. For example, they might assist a family and patient to decide if they wanted to refuse an intravenous tube or blood transfusion, which would provide a few more days of life but wouldn't cure the patient. The following account of a patient's decision not to pursue further diagnostic workups exemplifies the way providers of hospice care returned control to the patient.

When I returned [to Saint Christopher's Hospice] and discussed the matter I found we were all agreed that nothing should be done. Apparently clubbing or thickening of the finger-tips is one pointer to cancer of the lung, the blood supply being restricted, and since I had always been rather bronchitic it seemed quite likely that the primary might be there. I was told that if it was, nothing could be done and the information at this stage would merely be academic. It was pointless. It was not worth subjecting myself to things which made me uncomfortable or tired and unhappy. I was happy as I was. (Dunnet 1973)

**Interdisciplinary Team Approach** Hospice teams were interdisciplinary, and each member had equal status. Unlike illness, death cannot be "cured," so each staff member was considered of equal value in helping patient and family. Team members came from several professional groups, including the clergy, nurses, social workers, psychiatrists, and physicians. An unusual aspect of hospice teams was the importance accorded to the clergy. The hospice concept emphasized spiritual care; the intent was not to force religion on dying patients but to return spiritual services to terminal care.

Hospice philosophy also sought to blur professional roles, to humanize death, and to reduce the tendency among staff to fight over "who owns the body." Because terminal illness was a natural human experience, team members wanted to eliminate traditional status and authority roles. The team members pulled together and used their expertise to help the patient and family, and it was the patient and family who determined which team members would assist them.

Moreover, team members were available 24 hours a day. Hospice care providers wanted to alter the traditional medical practice of being available at the convenience of the staff rather than on the basis of patient or family need. Mrs. C., for example, had suffered from cancer for many months. She finally slipped into a coma, and it became apparent that she was dying. Her wish had been to die at home surrounded by family. The family wanted to honor Mrs. C.'s wish, but like many American families they had never witnessed a death, and they were frightened about what might occur. The hospice chaplain, nurse, and social worker helped them cope with their fears. The nurse was the first to arrive. She gently explained that Mrs. C.'s condition had deteriorated and that death seemed likely. The nurse did what was necessary to make Mrs. C. comfortable and explained as best she could what happens when someone dies. During the night she was relieved by the chaplain and social worker, who took turns helping the family cope with Mrs. C.'s impending death.

Finally, hospice care teams valued discussing their personal feelings about patients and fellow team members. According to hospice philosophy the workers' needs were important. The frustrations of working together, watching people die, and providing adequate care were discussed to ensure team members' effectiveness and to acknowledge that they, too, were affected by death.

**Pain Management and Symptom Control**  Hospice care represented not the end of treatment for the dying person but a different use of available technology. Pain management and symptom control include attending to the myriad physical causes of discomfort as well as the emotional and spiritual pain that contribute to patient and family distress during a terminal illness. Dr. Sylvia Lack, a student of Cicely Saunders and the first medical director at Hospice, Inc., stated that only 50 percent of cancer patients suffered from physical pain; much pain was the result of secondary consequences of their disease or of side effects from medical treatments. Anorexia, nausea, and constipation were examples of such problems.

Saunders avowed that no cancer patient need have pain if symptoms were properly assessed, and she established a variety of methods to fulfill this promise. Her methods for evaluating and treating physical discomfort integrated palliative support and modern medical technology (Saunders 1981, 96). Polypharmacy was the term Saunders used to describe her comprehensive approach to suffering. Pain was not just a physical sensation; it might be a consequence of loneliness, spiritual distress, inappropriate diet, or tumor growth. Careful listening was the most important skill in determining the best way to reduce patient discomfort. Interventions might be very simple, such as smoothing someone's brow while listening to him or her, or altering a patient's diet to reduce the constipating effects of most barbiturates.

The following case demonstrates how spiritual and psychological distress might be identified and treated through hospice care. Rose was a middle-aged woman with metastatic disease. Although physical pain was not typical to her illness, Rose complained of discomfort. Rather than ignoring her complaints or experimenting with different drug doses, the hospice team discussed the problem and hypothesized that pain might be her way of conveying her anxiety about the disease. To test their theory they used relaxation techniques to help Rose cope with anxiety. This method was effective. It helped Rose sleep at night and soothed her when she became lonely or anxious. Her complaints of pain subsided.

Palliative methods such as those described above were considered as important as sophisticated medical treatments, but they did not replace them. It is often thought that hospice care excludes the use of drugs, surgery, and other technologies. These treatments are used, but in the interest of comforting rather than curing. Thus radiation might be used to reduce tumor growth so that the patient has less pain or bleeding, or a tumor might be surgically removed if it prevents a patient from eating.

**Affordability** The final component of hospice care leaders envisioned early on was affordability. In fact, movement leaders believed it should be free. They argued that during the course of cancer illnesses people's financial resources were depleted, and that this compounded their stress. Therefore, hospice care providers believed that traditional reimbursement mechanisms and private philanthropies should fund programs. Like the British programs after which these initial U.S. programs were modeled, they used volunteers to supplement paid professionals. Thus, hospice programs with little financial support used trained volunteers to bathe patients, counsel families, and recommend palliative treatments.

## The First Three Programs

The first three modern American hospice programs were Hospice, Inc., Saint Luke's, and Hospice of Marin. These programs started with the same goals, but they differed in the form of care and the place of care. Hospice, Inc., and Hospice of Marin began as community-based programs emphasizing psychosocial support. Saint Luke's started in a teaching hospital and emphasized pain management and symptom control. Variations in form and emphasis established a pattern; programs altered their form and services to fit environments that were receptive to them. Hospice care providers encouraged these innovations, asserting that program idiosyncrasies reflected individual community needs.

**Hospice, Inc.** Founded by the Yale Study Group and located in Branford, Connecticut, Hospice, Inc., was the first American hospice to provide patient services. Based on Cicely Saunders's model of care, it was to be the only U.S. hospice to become a well-endowed institution with no ties to, or influence from, the acute health care system.

Rev. Edward Dobihal recalls the early years of Hospice, Inc., as a time of talking and endless meetings, which weren't without benefits. The hospice board was among the movement's minority constituency in its skepticism of the benefits of joining the acute health care system, and it resisted doing so. The board concluded that it did not want the hospice to be connected to the Yale University hospital. Members decided this for two reasons. First, they did not want to share funds with the hospital because this might adversely affect the hospice in times of financial strain. Second, they recognized that independence would protect them from value conflicts with acute health care providers (DuBois 1980). As a result, Hospice, Inc.'s, place in the movement's evolution is unique.

Following a series of lectures regarding death, dying, and hospice care at the Yale School of Nursing, Florence Wald, Rev. Dobihal, a minister at Yale/New Haven Hospital, and several other professionals from the Yale/New Haven community began meeting regularly. As Dobihal described it, "Those 1966 speakers raised our consciousness, but we were a group of loners, with different kinds of feelings. Some of us were angry about the lack of care or the incompetence; others were confused about what they were supposed to be doing" (Rossman 1977, 107). As the group, which in 1967 came to be called the Yale Study Group, continued meeting, it gradually focused on establishing hospices.

Wald received a grant in 1969 to study the needs of the dying patient. With the help of the Yale Study Group, she prepared and completed a report, "Interdisciplinary Study for Care of Dying Patients and Their Families," in 1971. The study found that dying people wanted health care that gave them comfort and that they wanted to die in their own homes. On the strength of these findings, a steering committee was established to look into developing a hospice program. That same year, members of the Yale Study Group became the board of directors of Hospice, Inc., an incorporated, nonprofit organization. The board obtained funding to employ staff for a hospice program serving the Yale/New Haven area.

Board members continued to carry out research projects to show the limitations of hospital environments for dying patients. For example, building on work by Glaser and Strauss (1965) and Kübler-Ross (1969), they conducted a participant observation study of terminal care in an acute care facility. Mimicking the symptoms of a dying patient, a member of the research team was admitted to a hospital, where staff relegated him to a back ward once they established that he was an unlikely candidate for cure. Their contact with him, as with his fellow dying patients, was brief and task oriented, making it difficult to ask questions about his condition (Buckingham, Lack, Mount, MacClean, and Collins 1976).

By 1973 Hospice, Inc., had enough community support and financing to begin providing home care services for terminally ill patients. As it happened, a visit by Saunders coincided with the board's decision to begin hiring staff, and she recommended a student of hers for the position of medical director. Consequently, Sylvia Lack became the first medical director of Hospice, Inc. Lack's first responsibility was to secure funding, and she went to Washington, D.C., to deliver a grant proposal to the National Cancer Institute (NCI).

Demonstration monies had become available to provide start-up funds for innovative health care programs, and hospice care was among the possible beneficiaries of these monies. In 1973 the NCI established a request for proposals to be submitted by groups that wanted to start hospices, but only Hospice, Inc., which had begun planning and development in 1971, was eligible. The $800,000 grant it received was a primary source of program support during its first years of service provision.

Although Hospice, Inc., started as a home care model, it did not stop at this juncture. Having received one NCI grant, it was quick to respond to NCI's second request for proposals in 1977. These funds and several other endowments from state and local funding sources were used to build a 44-person, inpatient facility in Branford. A few other facilities modeled themselves after Hospice, Inc., but their efforts to obtain financial support were less successful. Hospice, Inc.'s, separation from the acute health care system made it a bona fide institution, and it did not face the funding limitations experienced by other programs.

Hospice, Inc., is an anomaly in program development. Several factors explain this. First, it was the original hospice program and as such held a special position in the movement's history. Second, the board's decision to remove itself from other health care systems never wavered. Finally, Connecticut's governor, Eleanor Grasso, had a personal interest in hospice care. Grasso suffered from a cancer illness that eventually caused her death. While governor, she supported Hospice, Inc., by providing funds for its development and by supporting policies that legitimized hospice care as an alternative service. For example, in 1977 she allocated a $1.5 million grant to assist in building a separate hospice facility.

The board of Hospice, Inc., recognized the need to find public sources of support, and its administrator, Dennis Rezendes, hired in 1973, was adept at acquiring resources. In 1978, Hospice, Inc., became the first program approved for insurance reimbursement as a hospice home care service (Cohen 1979). And when the state of Connecticut allocated resources, Rezendes was quick to apply for matching federal funds.

When Medicare regulations were established in 1982, Hospice, Inc., received special consideration. Other hospice programs approved for Medicare benefits had to accept limited reimbursement for inpatient stays and for total cost of patient services. These restrictions did not apply to Hospice, Inc. According to Medicare regulations, any program that could prove it had begun services before 1975 was exempt from restrictions on inpatient stays and total cost of care. Only Hospice, Inc., which began its home care program in 1974, met this criterion.

Hospice, Inc., also took the lead in training others about hospice care. Rezendes and the other members of the Hospice, Inc., team shared their experiences with other groups who wanted to develop hospices. The first National Hospice Symposium, held in 1975, took place at Hospice, Inc. Seventy attendees representing 20 planning groups came to a two-day symposium where presenters, primarily members of Hospice, Inc., explained the principles of hospice care and the problems providers experienced as they started programs.

Hospice, Inc., obtained the trademark patent for the title *hospice* in 1976. They later relinquished it to the National Hospice Organization.

**Saint Luke's Hospice** The second hospice program in the United States was Saint Luke's. Developed at Saint Luke's Hospital, a teaching facility in New York City, it became the first of many hospital-based hospice programs. In fact, during the early years of program development, hospital-based programs were a popular program type.

The inspiration for Saint Luke's Hospice was Rev. Carlton Sweetser. In 1963 Sweetser was working as a chaplain at Sloan Kettering. This hospital was, and is, a cure-oriented cancer treatment center where patients are given the most advanced forms of therapy. Sloan Kettering was one stop on Saunders's 1963 lecture tour, and Sweetser heard her speak there. He was impressed by her concept of care and introduced himself to her. This was the start of a relationship that continued for many years. Following his introduction to the concept of hospice care Sweetser became an active participant in the death with dignity movement. He participated in the IWG, and he asserted the need for hospice services at the conferences sponsored by the Foundation of Thanatology.

He left Sloan Kettering Hospital and took a position as head chaplain at Saint Luke's. In the early 1970s he began his efforts to start a hospice program there. The way in which he finally got people to pay attention to his idea was unusual. Like any department head, as head chaplain he had to submit an annual report to the board of directors. Typically, such a report was a fairly standard and tedious document. On this occasion, however, Sweetser produced a lengthy appeal regarding the need for a hospice program at Saint Luke's Hospital. Much to his surprise and delight, his report attracted the attention of one of the board members, who contacted Sweetser and asked to be told more about hospices.

Sweetser eventually received the hospital board's approval to establish a program at Saint Luke's, and he assembled a hospice board, consisting of a social worker, nurse, radiologist, physician, and administrator. The funding and staff support necessary to start the program were easily obtained. The first major grant that Sweetser secured was $60,000 from the Episcopal Society of Women. This grant enabled the board to hire a full-time nurse and part-time medical director for the program. Other staff positions needed to complete the team were filled by volunteers from various hospital departments, and additional funds to support operating costs were obtained by holding fashion shows and luncheons. Saunders was an active participant in promoting this program's growth. She spoke at fund-raisers and helped acquire much needed funds.

The hospice boards' efforts to obtain a place for the program were not as successful. Funds raised through donations were not sufficient, and the hospital was unwilling to allocate space. Committed to having a hospice program, the board came up with a creative solution to the problem. They decided that if the hospital would not provide space, the team would go to the patients. A professional team trained in hospice care techniques visited patients at their bedsides and made recommendations about physical care to floor staff. Patients designated as hospice patients had special privileges, such as being allowed to have visitors at any time day or night or to visit a garden next to the hospital. This innovation in hospice care became known as the scatter-bed model, and its creation changed the definition of hospice from a place of care to a concept of care.

Saint Luke's integration with an acute health care hospital also influenced service delivery. As one team member described it, "We're working in a given situation. By that I mean we're working with a given staff, in a given facility. We're not starting fresh, with the ideal." As participants in an acute health care system, the team emphasized its expertise in pain management and symptom control. Because of funding limitations during their first years of operation, hospice care was available only from 9 A.M. to 5 P.M., five days a week, not around the clock.

At this stage of the movement's development, concerns about potential problems resulting from such an innovation were minimal. At the time, the hospice care team and the board had no intention of continuing to offer this kind of limited care; it was simply an expedient way to start a hospice program. But just as the separateness of Hospice, Inc., from acute care influenced its development and its future shape, Saint Luke's willingness to accommodate structural limitations remained a continuing problem. Saint Luke's Hospital was not interested in creating a separate hospice facility. The hospice team grew, their case load expanded, and they developed home care services, but they continued to visit patients wherever they were in the hospital.

Saint Luke's scatter-bed model was picked up by other program developers. Facilities that did not have sufficient staff or space imitated this program type. Saunders approved the model and introduced it to English facilities that suffered similar problems. This innovation had the potential to influence inpatient care, but it also tied the hospice program to the acute health care system. As research on the medical environment has shown, its values were not always sympathetic with attempts to humanize terminal care.

**Hospice of Marin**  Hospice of Marin in California was founded by William Lamers, a psychiatrist who experienced the emotional impact of death on families and friends when a close friend of his died. During his friend's illness he worked with the family, helping them to understand their loss. As noted previously, he initially wanted to develop a clinic where people could receive help with their grief reactions, but was convinced by Dr. Kübler-Ross to create a hospice program instead.

In 1974 he began meeting with a minister and a homemaker (his word) to develop a hospice. Over the next year community interest in the project increased. After completing an assessment of community need in 1975, the Hospice of Marin began providing in-home support services, but its staff was composed entirely of volunteers. This adaptation created a third program type, the volunteer community support team.

In late 1975 the decision was made to delay plans for development of an inpatient hospice facility and concentrate instead on delivering whatever services could be provided to a small number of patients, both to test the effectiveness of the hospice concept for care outside of an institution or facility, and to "develop a track record" that would provide experience for the hospice staff and evidence to the professional community of our intent to follow through on early planning. (Lamers 1978, 54)

Like Saint Luke's Hospice, Hospice of Marin initially hoped to some-day have an independent facility. But after observing other programs' failure to secure adequate funding for independent facilities, the board decided to incorporate the hospice as a home health agency.

Seeking legitimacy as a home health agency was a milestone in Hospice of Marin's development. In 1976 the board held a meeting to discuss ways to solve the overwhelming community demand for services. The board's solution was to expand and seek affiliation with the home health care system. Some had reservations about the effects of such a strategy on the program's ideals; would Hospice of Marin become just one more cold, impersonal medical bureaucracy, more concerned with meeting regulations than with providing individualized, humane care? Despite these concerns, the board resolved to become a formal organization and seek funds as a home health agency (Stoddard 1978).

Others who observed the work of the Hospice of Marin were convinced that the best way to provide hospice services was in patients' homes. Volunteer professionals and laypersons could participate in the provision of services, and this would keep the cost of services down. Hospice of North Carolina was one organization that was impressed by this argument and in the late 1970s set up a network of hospice home care services throughout North Carolina.

**Three Models of Care**   Each of these first three programs provided a different model of hospice care. This allowed for greater flexibility in starting new hospice programs, and as we can see from the case histories, once a model was established, it was institutionalized. Hospice, Inc., Saint Luke's Hospice, and Hospice of Marin also became educators. (Although Saint Christopher's Hospice in England continues to be "the place" to learn methods of hospice care.) Groups that wanted to develop hospice programs could visit each and learn about its service method. In 1976 Rev. Dobihal reported receiving 36 requests for such assistance (DuBois 1980). Hospice of Marin and Saint Luke's Hospice also received their share of requests, and these providers had to establish ways to cope with all the visitors. They established training programs, complete with slides and print materials to explain their model of hospice care. Hospice, Inc., and Hospice of Marin hired a staff person to conduct the training. Visits to Saint Luke's were restricted to one day a week so that patient care would not be disrupted.

## Resistance to Hospice Care

Not every group that attempted to create a hospice program succeeded. Hospice supporters claimed that hospice programs were a desired change; in actuality, there was a great deal of resistance to them. This resistance, however, never coalesced into formal attempts to stop the hospice movement. It was evidenced by a variety of criticisms.

Hospice care was criticized because its emphasis on death might inhibit a patient's fight for life. Lofland (1978) called it the "happy death movement" and stated that "an accepted solution resolves a problem but it also reduces the availability of alternative solutions. If the 'natural death' philosophy comes to dominate medical practice, for example, the individual who wants to use every conceivable medical technology to prolong his or her life regardless of cost or efficacy becomes the odd person out" (Spiegel 1983, 136).

Hospice care was also criticized for its integration with the larger health care system. Melvin Krant, a supporter of Saunders's concept of hospice care, predicted its demise in the United States. "It's going to fail as an American idea. It will get into operation but its content will fail," because it will further fragment the overspecialized medical industry (Holden 1978, 390).

Reactions to hospice care at Strong Memorial Hospital in Rochester, New York, exemplify the resistance hospice proponents sometimes encountered in trying to start programs. A physician at this hospital who believed that the cure-oriented nature of medical care was detrimental to some patients wanted to introduce the hospice concept to the hospital's services. He began planning for such a program in 1973 and finally obtained funding to support a needs study in 1975, but support for the project "had always been soft. Many hospital personnel simply had not been sold on the desirability of a hospice before they were asked to contribute to it" (DuBois 1980, 131). For a year the hospital employed a staff person whose job it was to establish the need for a hospice program, but her position was abruptly terminated, ostensibly because the funds had run out. Anecdotal reports indicated that the staff disliked this person's work with patients. It was suggested that she had alienated staff. Personality disputes might have been one reason the program was not well received, but an overall assessment of this program's failure by those directly involved found that hospital personnel were uncomfortable with the hospice concept and therefore uncomfortable with the staff member's attempts to talk about dying.

Funding limitations were another impediment to hospice programs' development. For example, at Saint Joseph's Hospital in New York a group of professionals formed a hospice board in 1977. By the following year the group had disbanded, and plans for a hospice program were scrapped. The pastoral care department, headed by a clergywoman, had initiated the formation of a planning board of hospital staff who were interested in the hospice concept. Staff members who supported the idea met regularly, but hospital administrators did not participate. When approached by the hospice board, the administration refused to fund such a project; administrators expressed objection to the plan was that hospice programs did not have a reliable source of revenue.

As we can see from the above examples, the concept of hospice care was not without critics. But these individuals continued to be just that, individuals, not members of a concerted countereffort. They did prevent the development of some programs, but overall the movement continued to gain political and popular support.

## The Culmination of the Coalescent Stage

Innovation changed the definition of *hospice* from a facility where one received special services to a concept of care that could be provided anywhere. Providers referred to this structural change as "hospice the adjective, not the noun." Traditionally, hospices were associated with buildings or institutions, usually run by religious groups. Patients went to such facilities to receive care during their final days. Modern hospice programs were not established in special buildings; they were conceived as a method of care that could be provided in a variety of settings, even the patient's home. This evolution in the definition of hospice programs was not without problems. The public became confused as to what service hospice offered. Such confusion persists in the 1990s: terminally ill people and their families seek out hospices as if they were places to spend the last days of life only to find out that families will have to assume responsibility for care at home, with the help of hospice staff.

Although Saint Luke's Hospice and the Hospice of Marin are credited as being the second and third programs, many groups established hospice services during this time. By 1976, 36 groups were providing or planning to provide hospice care in the United States. These groups were located in metropolitan areas in several states, including California, New York, Pennsylvania, Florida, Illinois, Missouri, and Arizona. Developers might be an individual minister wanting to start a local volunteer group, a group at a hospital wanting to mimic the Saint Luke's model, or a group hoping to create an independent facility.

The following statement by a speaker at the second National Hospice conference, held in 1977 in Riverside, New Jersey, demonstrates the strong desire, but limited resources, early providers had to help dying patients.

> Saint Barnabas is composed entirely of women from the community and we are located in a small Episcopal church. We have no office, no phones except my kitchen phone, and we have no money. We help primarily as facilitator; lay people to help bring about better care in the institutions that are already in our country. Our program consists of two parts, education and volunteer visitors. We speak to community organizations like the PTA or a local nursing home staff, and we visit terminally patients referred to us on a regular basis.

Establishing different programs forms was possible given the diverse beliefs of the participants, but it also encouraged deflection from ideals. The earliest creators of hospices believed that the movement's popularity would prevail over structural limitations, but programs that imitated Saint Luke's or the Hospice of Marin were not as firm in their belief that hospice care should take place in a separate facility. These developers saw no reason not to maintain their chosen form of service. Inpatient hospice programs believed that this was the best way to provide terminally ill patients with alternative care, and home care advocates were equally firm that their form of service was the ideal model.

These first programs attempted to provide a full complement of hospice services, but structural differences resulted in variations in the way services were provided. On the one hand, home care hospice programs' ability to influence pain control methods or to maintain continuity of care when a patient required hospitalization was limited. On the other hand, programs affiliated with hospitals placed less emphasis on talking about dying and providing bereavement support services following the death of a patient.

## Conclusion

Conflicting ideologies dominated the hospice movement during its coalescence. From its inception, the diversity of beliefs among the participants, as well as their limited power, affected the course of the movement. Advocates of hospice care were largely ministers, nurses, and survivors. Their enthusiasm made it popular among people and professionals like themselves, but this constituency lacked the political power necessary to fully implement its ideals, and it had limited access to the financial resources that would have allowed for independence. As a result, hospice care providers had to be adaptable. This was one of the movement's greatest assets in allowing it to go forward, but was one of its greatest shortcomings in allowing the co-optation of its ideals.

*Chapter 6*

# The Peak of the Movement

Interest in hospice care by the American public and health care providers peaked during the early part of the 1980s. Conferences, publications, and organizations proliferated as participants clamored to learn more about the concept of hospice care. One organization, the National Hospice Organization, represented the political interests of the movement. Its members emphasized legitimizing hospice programs as a health care service. The number of programs increased; some were similar to the first three models, but many were not. Although enthusiasm to start programs was high, funding was limited, and hospice developers continued to adapt programs to fit whatever environment would support their existence; ultimately six program types were created.

Concomitantly, politicians, medical entrepreneurs, and policymakers became interested in hospice care. Liberal politicians were attracted by hospice leaders' claims that they were initiating humanitarian reform of terminal care; medical entrepreneurs saw hospices as a potentially profitable extension of the health care industry; and policymakers believed it would reduce health care costs. The older leaders of the movement, often characterized as "impractical idealists," suggested a cautious approach to such interest, but the directors of the newly formed NHO and medical entrepreneurs who administered new hospice programs encouraged the attentions of policymakers.

As the majority of hospice providers integrated with health care systems the services they offered changed; services were redefined based on medical values, and much of what had made hospice care unique—such as bereavement counseling or spiritual services—was not

108

encouraged in traditional medical environments. In 1982 Medicare established a hospice benefit. This reimbursement reflected policymakers' bias toward cost-efficient health care.

By the early 1980s core members observed the negative impact that reimbursement and affiliation with the health care systems had on programs. By seeking federal dollars "reform groups were forced into tight corners where they sought rescue by institutions that might or might not have their best interests at heart" (Foster, Wald, and Wald 1978, 24). To gain sanction, hospice advocates joined the medical system; they did not fight it. Contrary to leaders' claims, the hospice movement, rather than reforming medical care, added a new concept: treatment of the terminally ill. Hospice programs were considered to be an alternative health care benefit, but in form they resembled traditional medical settings with hospice overtones (Dooley 1982). Programs became a middle ground between allowing someone to die without treatment and using every machine and method possible to delay death.

These events are typical to the institutional stage of a social movement, as described by Mauss. He predicts that during this phase a movement achieves its greatest popular success. Simultaneously, alterations in the movement's aims occur as leaders compromise goals to acquire resources and support from external political forces. Participation also shifts. New leaders are attracted to the movement, but they are motivated to join the movement out of self-interest and they espouse goals that are incongruous with the movement's ideals. These new leaders do not pretend to support the original ideals of the movement; they may even criticize such goals as unrealistic.

## Hospice: A Popular Concept

By the late 1970s the hospice movement had achieved national renown. Articles on hospice care appeared in national publications such as *Newsweek*, *Cosmopolitan*, the *New York Times*, the *Wall Street Journal* and the *Washington Star*. There were televised commercials about hospice's benefits, and Jack Klugman became the movement's celebrity spokesperson. Numerous books and publications—later characterized as reiterative to the point of being noninformative (Butterfield-Picard and Magno 1982)—described the development and importance of the hospice movement (Cohen 1979; Davidson 1978; Lack and Buckingham 1978; Rossman 1977; Stoddard 1978).

In 1976 the Library of Congress included *hospice* in its glossary of terms, and in 1979 it became a separate category in the *Index Medicus*. Newsletters were created to update providers and the public about program achievements and legislation affecting hospice care. Hospice, Inc., obtained a grant supporting publication of such a newsletter and in 1976 reported a list of 3,500 subscribers. Hillhaven Hospice, in Tucson, Arizona, published a similar newsletter.

Many politicians offered their support. Sen. Jennings Randolph, whose wife had died from cancer and who experienced the isolation and stress of caregiving without much support, asserted the importance of federal support for care (1982). Sen. Edward Kennedy, a supporter of government-sponsored health care services, agreed to give the opening address at the first National Hospice Meeting in Washington, D.C., in 1982. That same year President Ronald Reagan designated a week in November as National Hospice Week, thus recognizing the hospice movement as an important social cause. Subsequently, November was designated National Hospice Month.

## Annual Conferences
## and a National Hospice Organization

As more people became interested in creating programs, they sought training in the principles of hospice care and in the "how tos" of program start-up. Symposiums were arranged to meet these demands. During 1977 three national conferences, large formal versions of earlier attempts to spread the word about hospice, were held. The first of these conferences took place at Riverside Hospice in New Jersey, followed by a second at Hospice of Marin in California, and a third at Hospice, Inc., in Connecticut. In 1978 the fervor to learn about hospice care continued, and two more national conferences were held, the National Conference of Social Welfare and the First Annual National Hospice Organization Symposium. Conference attendance also increased: in 1975 a training seminar at Hospice, Inc., had only 70 attendees; by 1978, when NHO held its first annual conference in Washington, D.C., more than 1,000 people attended (Wald 1983). By attending a hospice symposium, one could learn about the techniques of hospice care, the way a hospice group had approached state or local authorities for funds, the difficulties providers had obtaining community support, and/or the opposition the hospice concept encountered from the medical community.

A constant theme at national conferences was the need for insurance dollars to support hospice programs. The majority of providers believed that to survive they must seek health care dollars, as if this were the only way to maintain hospice programs. They feared that fund-raising and foundation grants would be insufficient to sustain their services (Holden 1978). There was a minority constituency of skeptics who voiced doubts about integration with the health care system, but their voices were stilled by the majority who wanted hospice to become a legitimate adjunct to the health care industry.

Although this strategy was incongruous with the movement's early ideals and some movement leaders believed it unwise to seek insurance reimbursement, this pursuit gave the movement a clarity of purpose that it had lacked. The movement became politically unified as the majority of hospice leaders agreed to pursue legislation making hospice care an alternative benefit under the Medicare program.

Such meetings also brought together movement leaders, giving them the opportunity to form an organization empowered to promote the ideals of hospice care nationally, to develop standards for existing hospice services, and to pursue the legitimization of hospice care. At the second national conference hospice leaders formed a committee to explore the need for a national organization. (The Hospice National Advisory Council, mentioned earlier, was not made up of hospice providers. Council members had the power and influence to give the movement clout with legislators; they did not participate in establishing funds or regulating hospice services. Therefore another organization was developed to organize hospice providers.) A task force headed by Charlotte Shedd of the Buffalo Hospice Program outlined the purpose for such an agency: to educate the public about hospice care, to integrate hospice care with the acute health care system, and to find funding sources. The committee also wanted to seek funds without compromising ideals. Members asserted that a national organization should represent all movement participants. They proposed a sliding-scale membership fee so that struggling programs with little funding could participate along with the better-endowed hospital-based programs.

At the third symposium the above committee, known as the Hospice Organization Committee, was renamed the National Hospice Organization and by-laws and an executive board were established. Zachory P. Morfogen, chair of Riverside Hospice's Board of Directors, was NHO's first chair, and Dennis Rezendes, the administrator of Hospice, Inc., its first executive secretary. During the next two years what had started as little more than a desire for an organization became a functioning political structure. NHO incorporated and opened offices in Washington, D.C. Josefina Magno became its first executive director.

Magno writes of her initiation to NHO, "At Georgetown Hospital I received a call, 'Will you please be the program director for the first annual meeting of the national hospice organization?' Fool that I was, I said yes. The caller said the meeting was to be in Washington, D.C., because our national leaders should know about hospice. I soon discovered there was no national hospice organization, there was no money, there was nothing" (Magno 1990, 114).

Although NHO's mandate was to represent all hospice interests, attention to funding soon outweighed other concerns. Created to educate and regulate a developing hospice industry, NHO soon assumed the role of public relations representative to medical providers and third-party insurers. Early on leaders disagreed about NHO's goals, and during the late 1970s a splinter group called the National Education Project attempted to lobby for Medicare funding for hospice care. This group rejoined NHO as the latter organization, too, focused on obtaining Medicare/Medicaid support (Paradis and Cummings 1986).

"If hospice care is to be integrated appropriately into the fabric of the nation's health care delivery system, organizations of the various medical and health care professionals and providers must collaborate to assure that hospice care in this country does not fall victim of American faddism. The dynamic NHO leadership increases the prospect of early recognition of hospice care as a reimbursable modality option" (Hackley 1979, 53). In particular, Donald Gaetz, an executive officer of NHO, focused on obtaining reimbursement for hospice programs; years later providers charged that in doing so he had compromised hospice philosophy.

Hospice care providers did not enthusiastically embrace NHO. NHO was a strong lobbyist for hospice care, but by 1982 only half the existing hospice programs had become members. Attempts to standardize hospice care and seek insurance reimbursement regardless of the deleterious effects on the nature of the care were discouraging to many who joined the movement. The majority of the movement's leaders, however, favored reimbursement, and participants who disagreed rarely asserted their objections; it was only in hindsight that providers complained. As the negative impact of Medicare reimbursement began to be felt by all participants, those who had disagreed with the movement's political course complained that a few powerful groups had been allowed to speak for everyone.

State and local hospice boards were also created to assert the legitimacy of hospice care as an alternative health care system and to obtain program funding. In California, Connecticut, and New York hospice boards formed and *attempted* to standardize programs by establishing criteria for program services and staff. (Use of the term *attempt* is deliberate. As we'll see, hospice providers tended to resist all efforts to standardize services, even when it meant losing funding eligibility.) In other states, local groups such as the Southeastern Wisconsin Hospice Council, representing a portion of the state's hospice programs, sought legitimacy and obtain funding for their members. For example, this latter group convinced the United Auto Workers Union in that area to endorse hospice benefits for its members.

## The Rise of Programs

Despite the lack of any hard evidence proving their benefits (Osterweiss and Champagne 1978), hospice programs flourished during the early 1980s. The U.S. Government Accounting Office's characterization of programs is the most accurate one. "There is no standard definition of what a hospice is or what services an organization must provide to be considered a hospice" (1979, 1). As programs proliferated tolerance for program innovation persisted; new programs were chameleon-like, adapting to the environment in which they developed. Variation in form permitted program developers to gravitate somewhat arbitrarily toward or away from the movement's ideals. Some providers emphasized treatments whereas others stressed psychosocial support.

Initially, independent hospice facilities were the preferred hospice model, but funding was difficult to obtain. Hospice leaders were wary of affiliation with hospitals, believing that hospital administrators who wanted to fill empty beds would accept hospice programs and then interfere with the provision of services. Policymakers, however, were hesitant to build new inpatient facilities, believing it fiscally irresponsible. Improvements in health care services, changes in insurance coverage, and the expansion of long-term care facilities had reduced hospital bed use.

Therefore, despite their concern about the dangers of integrating with hospitals, many providers did so. In fact, during the late 1970s hospital-based programs were the most popular model; by 1980, 46 percent of all hospice programs were affiliated with hospitals. Ultimately, program form was shaped by funding as hospice leaders adapted to funding restrictions.

**The First National Funding for Hospice Care** To give the hospice care concept a trial the National Cancer Institute planned to support about six programs for a period of three years. But its support was halfhearted. Many who participated in NCI's hearings regarding the viability of hospice services were convinced that hospices would be grim places where people went to die. Lawrence Burke, an NCI spokesman, announced that hospice care should be given a fair trial, but applicants were restricted by red tape and time limitations (Davidson 1978). Moreover, NCI refused to fund hospital-based programs, the most popular form of program. NCI agreed with those hospice advocates who asserted that hospital philosophy was contradictory to hospice philosophy and that hospitals would create hospice programs simply to fill unused beds (Holden 1978).

In 1977 NCI awarded grants to Hospice, Inc., in Connecticut, Kaiser Permanente in Norwalk, California, Hillhaven Hospice in Tucson, and Riverside Hospice in New Jersey. These were to be the last monies allocated to develop hospice facilities. Policymakers decided that the cost of creating independent facilities' was prohibitive, thus short-circuiting efforts to recreate the Saint Christopher's model in America. The four independent hospice programs that were supported by this funding became the only independent hospice facilities for cancer patients in this country. (The term *freestanding*, frequently used in the hospice literature, is misleading. It refers to community programs that are not affiliated with larger health care systems. These programs do not maintain independent inpatient facilities.)

Further proof of the power of unsubstantiated claims made by social movement leaders was found in the way that NCI funded demonstration projects without stipulating what constituted a program or what it should accomplish. "Although we agree that evaluation is necessary, neither NCI nor Hospice, Inc., [is] sure . . . how an evaluation should be done" (Hospice, Inc., 1976). It was not until 1978, following NCI's funding of three other demonstration grants, that these hospices, along with NCI, determined what should be evaluated. They established four research areas: first, did pharmaceutical and advanced clinical techniques ease physical discomfort; second, does the supportive environment of hospice ease patient and family psychological discomfort; third, does hospice care sustain patient and family emotional stability; and fourth, what are the benefits of this multidisciplinary approach that go beyond the traditional medical model?

**Program Proliferation: How Great Was It?** During the late 1970s popular interest in hospice care was greater than program growth. The tendency to overstate the number of programs served an obvious function; it encouraged participants to view their reform efforts as successful and it supported the belief that hospice was a popularly desired alternative to the acute health care system. Although 33 states had hospice societies, few programs existed (Breindel and Boyle 1979). "The exposure of the American public to the hospice concept through lectures, seminars, workshops, and community meetings is great when compared with the actual number of patients and families being cared for in this country, within the framework of a realistic hospice philosophy. That there is deception is indicated by the fact that there are extremely few hospice beds available and few ongoing hospice home care services" (Klagsbrun 1983, 23).

According to hospice advocates there were about 47 hospice programs by the end of 1976 (Faulkner and Kugler 1981), whereas by May 1978 hospice sources suggested there were 165 programs in 33 states (Breindel and Boyle 1979). According to Cohen (1979), approximately 220 programs were in various stages of development around 1979. The U.S. Government Accounting Office (1979), however, in a national survey conducted in 1978, found only 59 programs. Using established listings and providers' reports, GAO researchers made more than 500 inquiries to facilities or groups providing or planning to provide hospice services during the period July to September 1978. They found only 59 programs that offered at least one hospice service and 73 other groups that were planning or attempting to plan a program.

Hospice care providers also misused some information. Cohen listed four programs in the New York state area as being under development, but they never materialized. He also listed places such as Calvary Hospital and Rosary Hill. These facilities had existed since the turn of the century, and Calvary Hospital is a specialty hospital, not a hospice. Official listings such as those compiled by state hospice associations also included potential providers, and few efforts were made to update program status. Russell (1985) contacted 200 programs listed by NHO and state health care rosters and found that several had never provided services or had ceased to provide such services.

The first sign of actual program proliferation was the result of the Medicare demonstration projects, which began in 1980. The Joint Commission on Accreditation for Hospitals in 1981 found 440 programs providing hospice services and another 560 in various stages of planning. Of the 440 existing programs, 51 percent had developed after 1980

(Faulkner and Kugler 1981). By 1984 NHO found 935 programs providing hospice care and another 400 groups planning a program.

**A Political Opportunity**　Many factors encouraged participant enthusiasm for the hospice care concept, but it was a political opportunity that
led to program proliferation. As health care costs rose at a pace faster than
inflation, policymakers sought ways to reduce these costs, particularly
those incurred during the last weeks of life. Terminal care as provided by
hospice programs emphasized palliative care and death at home; therefore
it had the potential to reduce costs.

Rumors began to circulate in 1976 that federal officials were considering funding hospice programs. Appeals from Sens. Kennedy, Ribicoff,
and Robert Dole for information about hospice care further reinforced the
belief that providers were approaching a time when hospice care would
become reimbursed as a separate form of service. The idea that hospices
cut costs was not new, but it gained favor as more hospice providers
agreed that integrating with the health care system was "the way" to stim-
ulate program growth. Before 1977 assertions about hospice care emphasized the emotional and physical benefits that providers accomplished.
After 1977 descriptions of hospice care included the statement, "and
hospice is cost-effective."

In 1978 Joseph Califano, director of the Department of Health, Education, and Welfare, announced at the October National Hospice Organization meeting that a two-year hospice demonstration project would be
funded by Medicare and Medicaid. Simultaneously, Blue Cross/Blue
Shield suggested that it, too, was interested in supporting demonstration
projects. Demonstration periods would establish hospice care's benefits
and ability to reduce costs. In 1978 the Health Care Financing Administration invited applications for Medicare demonstration projects. In all, 26
sites were chosen, and providers were expected to sign agreements during
fiscal year 1979; the actual project did not begin until 1980, however.
Similarly, Blue Cross/Blue Shield invited programs to participate in a
demonstration project that also began in 1980.

Hospice programs that participated in demonstration projects received
unrestricted financial support. During the demonstration period these
hospices were funded for all services, and insurers waived many of their
restrictions for atypical services, such as bereavement counseling,
extended in-home palliative support, and inpatient respite care. Hospice
providers and medical entrepreneurs who observed the way that demonstration projects were funded assumed that these exemptions would

continue when hospice care became an approved benefit of insurers. Many new programs were developed based on the premise that hospice care's future as an adequately funded service was assured.

**Hospice Care Is Cheaper** Claims of low costs were part of the movement's rhetoric. They were never proved (Aiken and Marx 1982). Hospice services were inexpensive in that they made little use of technology, but they were expensive because they had high patient/staff ratios. Moreover, different program types incurred different costs. When the GAO (1979) conducted its study of hospice services, it reported that no assessment could be made of costs because there were no accurate data on types or quantity of services offered to patients and families.

Despite differences in the way programs provided services and limited evaluation of costs, assertions that hospice care was cheaper than hospital care were common. A hospice program in Washington, D.C., assessed its costs at $160 a day, half the cost of hospital care in that area. Hospice of Columbus in Ohio estimated its cost per patient at $65 per day, whereas the hospital cost was $126 per day. The Genesee Home Care Association studied its New York programs and found that the actual cost of care for 55 patients over a period of 1,576 days was $118,626. Physicians estimated that the cost of acute care for these same patients for only 943 days would have been $212,175 (Buckingham, 1983).

In contrast, other data suggested that hospice in its pure form was not low in cost. "In England, the per-patient cost is about 80 percent of that in general hospital, and about 85 percent of the budget goes to staff salaries" (Cohen 1979, 86). Although patients in American hospice programs received little in the way of expensive testing, they received care for twice as long (Cohen 1979). The NCI demonstration projects found that hospice costs varied widely, and these costs were no less expensive than existing services. Nevertheless, assertions that hospice was cheaper persisted; as with much of the information about hospice care, speculative or short-term data were frequently accepted as facts.

**The Vicissitudes of Program Development** Government funding encouraged program growth, but to survive program developers had to adapt program structure; providers were creative, implementing hospice care in whatever setting they could. In addition to the first three hospice models, previously described, three other models of care became popular: a separate hospital floor or wing with its own staff trained in hospice techniques; a case management program that provided counseling services for patients and families but did not provide direct physical care; and a home care program that was part of an established home health care agency, such as the Visiting Nurse Service. During the late 1970s hospital-based programs were the most common form, but as the Medicare law was enacted the trend in program form shifted toward a home health care model.

All but one of the six different program types were affiliated with traditional health care systems. As feared by some hospice leaders, integration with the health care industry resulted in physicians and medical entrepreneurs redefining hospice services to compensate for staff shortages, discharge problems, and high health care costs. Not all hospice providers chose this medicalized version of care; some, particularly older, volunteer community programs, persisted in their attempts to demedicalize the dying process. Volunteer community programs, however, had a low profile. In these programs the movement's humanistic ideals were preserved, but they did not receive the publicity that hospital-based programs did, nor did they influence the political course of the movement.

Hospice programs are categorized into six types, but these types were anything but uniform. "Hospice programs in the United States are very individualized. Although they share a basic conceptual approach, they differ in setting, service components, reimbursement arrangements, and staffing. Each seems to evolve out of the needs and resources of its own community" (Osterweiss and Champagne 1979, 494). Klagsbrun stated, "We have reached the age of procreation, spawning other hospices, who like children, are often quite different from ourselves" (1983, 5). The institutions in which hospice units were located varied; hospitals, nursing homes, or VA hospitals might be a choice for an inpatient unit, with one bed or ten for hospice patients. Some even mixed terminally ill cancer patients in units with patients who suffered from other chronic diseases.

One program provided inpatient hospice services at a psychiatric facility. Klagsbrun (1983) described this unit, suggesting that hospice providers were not trained in psychiatry and therefore felt ill-equipped to cope with mentally ill patients who also were terminally ill; providing hospice care in a psychiatric facility made such services accessible to this population. Moreover, psychiatric staff were predisposed to hospice work because they were accustomed to spending their time talking with patients and because psychiatrists were accustomed to using barbiturates around the clock to control symptoms.

The case management hospice program might involve a minister who had a few volunteers and a lot of contact with health care agencies, or it might involve a large community group consisting of clergy, nurses, physicians, social workers, and lay people who provided emotional support for families who requested hospice services. Another example of the case management model was a hospital based program that oversaw rather than provided direct services for patients. At a California hospital the administration, bowing to pressure from its nursing department, assigned one nurse to implement hospice philosophy with selected patients throughout the hospital. This nurse oversaw patient care, made suggestions regarding ways to position or feed patients that provided them greater comfort, and helped families understand the physical processes that occurred as patients' conditions deteriorated.

Hospice programs associated with a home health agency might have a completely autonomous staff or might use home care staff to offer hospice care to certain patients. One home care program within a community home health agency had a separate coordinator, a minister, and a part-time social worker who worked only with hospice patients. Other staff members, such as nurses, home health aides, and physical therapists, were shared with the home health agency. Therefore, staff nurses had acutely ill, chronically ill, and terminally ill patients on their caseloads.

During the late 1970s the inspiration for new hospice programs continued to come from individuals who wanted to improve conditions for dying patients. Cabrini Hospice in New York, for example, was inspired by a chaplain at Cabrini Hospital. Father Pulciano, a Catholic priest who suffered from cancer, created a hospice program in a convent adjacent to the hospital. This program was one of the first hospice programs to combine a separate hospital unit with home care services. In California Elisabeth Kübler-Ross, who offered her services free, opened a teaching center, Shanti Nilaya, in 1977. This facility, based on a volunteer model, was a place of retreat that promoted psychological, physical, and spiritual healing for patients and families.

As different program types were imitated and proliferated, leaders of the hospice movement affirmed the benefits of their innovations. Hospice programs should meet community needs, not some bureaucratic standard, and leaders opposed preserving one form of hospice service over another. Developers "must not obscure their vision of hospice with buildings, or develop an 'edifice' complex. Inpatient units are helpful as backup for the home-care program and offer an alternative for some patients, but a hospice program can begin without a building" (Buckingham 1983, 66). Others suggested that only a few independent hospice centers were needed. These centers would serve as models of hospice care and would train new providers, while the majority of programs would consist of small groups of individuals working separately or within existing health care settings.

By the early 1980s, however, the expansion of medical services dominated hospice care. Hospital and home care administrators created hospice programs because they added a new service and increased their census. The staff they employed brought with them a belief in the hospice movement's mission, but their idealism was contained by the bureaucratic demands of the system that hired them. For example, emphasis was placed on making sure that patients complied with medical routines, even though individual staff members might believe that such treatments did little to improve the patient's quality of life.

Incorporation with medical settings resulted in the restriction of some aspects of hospice care, such as spiritual and bereavement support. Facilitating the reduction of these services was the emphasis by some providers on physical support. If care of physical needs was met, it was believed, patients' emotional needs would take care of themselves (Lack and Buckingham 1978). This view was frequently promoted in training and recruiting new participants, and it was further encouraged by the fact that services emphasizing physical care survived, whereas programs emphasizing psychosocial support did not (Buckingham and Lupu 1982). Predictably, medically oriented programs were over represented and their values dominated movement politics.

## Leaders Attempt to Define Program
## Services and Goals

Standards for hospice care emerged as a way to regulate the services provided by hospice programs and to facilitate access to health care funding. The popular interest in death and dying, the underutilization of hospital beds, and the rapid spread of program types aroused concern among leaders that without standards for hospice care services, the concept might be misused. Furthermore, having so many different program forms while having no regulations about what constituted adequate service provision inhibited hospice providers' consideration as an acceptable medical alternative.

The newly formed National Hospice Organization decided that establishing standards for hospice care would place providers in a better position to promote the hospice concept and to form liaisons with the Joint

Commission on Accreditation of Hospitals and other health organizations. In 1979, the International Work Group on Death, Dying, and Bereavement published assumptions of hospice principles. NHO, using these assumptions, published the first official standards for hospice care (see figure 1).

NHO's effort to develop standards "was met by providers with hostility, resistance, and widespread disbelief that standards were necessary" (Tehan 1985, 11). The majority of providers wanted to preserve hospice's idiosyncratic qualities, and they refused to accept standards. Flexibility of form was a strong and valued concept within the movement; program differences were important, providers said, because they permitted hospice developers to adapt to the needs of local communities. The restrictions inherent to standards would "rob" the movement of its idealism and innovation (Crowther 1980).

The standards set by NHO did not acknowledge the small volunteer programs that emphasized psychosocial support, nor did they accept medically oriented programs that did not have strong volunteer components. The movement's participants did not want to restrict individuals, however different their ideas, from being part of the movement. Said differently, any system that provided some aspect of hospice philosophy was welcome. Programs like Saint Luke's, which favored credible medical care, had as much claim to call themselves hospice as did community volunteer programs, such as the Maine Hospice Program, which provided only psychosocial support. Both kinds of programs were valued, but both provided different services.

During this phase of the movement we can see further evidence of the impact of an ideology derived from contradictory perspectives. Leaders had opposing viewpoints. As programs varied in the way they implemented hospice philosophy, leaders differed in the way they reacted to the integration of hospice care with traditional medical care. Health care workers who conceived of hospice care as a way to make "good death" possible shared leadership with medical entrepreneurs, newcomers to the movement who saw hospice care as a way to expand the health care industry.

Despite their conflicting values and ideas, leaders attempted to coexist. Everyone wanted hospice programs to proliferate, but differed in what they wanted to accomplish. At one extreme were leaders who wanted to go slowly to preserve hospice's unique character. At the other extreme were those who asserted that the time was right for hospice care to take its place in the acute health care system.

# Figure 1 Standards of a Hospice Program of Care

1. The hospice program complies with applicable local, state, and federal law and regulation governing the organization and delivery of health care to patients and families.
2. The hospice program provides a continuum of inpatient and home care services through an integrated administrative structure.
3. The home care services are available 24 hours a day, seven days a week.
4. The patient/family is the unit of care.
5. The hospice program has admission criteria and procedures that reflect:
    a. the patient/family's desire and need for service.
    b. physician participation.
    c. diagnosis and prognosis.
6. The hospice program seeks to identify, teach, coordinate, and supervise persons to give care to patients who do not have a family member available.
7. The hospice program acknowledges that each patient/family has its own beliefs and/or value system and is respectful of them.
8. Hospice care consists of a blending of professional and nonprofessional services, provided by an interdisciplinary team, including a medical director.
9. Staff support is an integral part of the hospice program.
10. Inservice training and continuing education are offered on a regular basis.
11. The goal of hospice care is to provide symptom control through appropriate palliative therapies.
12. Symptom control includes assessing and responding to the physical, emotional, social, and spiritual needs of the patient/family.
13. The hospice program provides bereavement services to survivors for a period of at least one year.
14. There will be a quality assurance program that includes:
    a. evaluation of services.
    b. regular chart audits.
    c. organizational review.
15. The hospice program maintains accurate and current integrated records on all patient/families.
16. The hospice complies with all applicable state and federal regulations.
17. The hospice inpatient unit provides space for:
    a. patient/family privacy.
    b. visitation and viewing.
    c. food preparation by the family.

*Source:* National Hospice Organization.

Those opposed to participating in the acute health care system recommended deliberateness of purpose and separation from outside influence as the prudent course. Hospital practice was the antithesis of hospice practice (Cohen 1979). Remaining autonomous from the health care system would preserve hospice care's integrity and originality (Dobihal 1974). Social policy that regulated hospice care might affect it adversely by making hospice services fit the traditional health care mold before its innovative, informal, and supportive components were in place.

Giving the keynote address at a meeting of hospice providers, John Hackley stated, "Given the carrot of possible reimbursement and the fashionable appeal of the subject of death and dying, the potential for misuse of the hospice philosophy and concept is obviously high" (National Conference on Social Welfare 1978, 3). Furthermore, utilizing health care systems to spread programs, one pessimist suggested, might result in "Kentucky Fried Hospice"—a hospice franchise that could be developed anywhere and would be exploited by hospital administrators who needed to utilize empty beds.

Kübler-Ross expressed the idealists' sentiment when she stated, "We need to go slowly, to become very selective in the choosing of the sites and especially the staff. We have to put competition and monetary or political interest aside and work in the spirit of Mother Teresa, to serve our fellow man regardless of any other issues" (Ewens and Herrington 1983, part 1).

Moderating these views were those leaders who accepted that participation in the acute health care system would fund programs adequately, but they recommended that such integration occur slowly. Wald suggested that "communication and working relationships between idealists and policymakers are necessary to keep the reform viable. That is a crucial point in the hospice movement in the United States. Inherent in all these reforms is an adversary position with regard to existing systems. Reformers are faced with the reactions their ideals cause on institutions with a vested interest in the status quo" (1983, 20).

Cautionary voices, however, were overshadowed by optimists and entrepreneurs who asserted that the time was right for program development and that to succeed hospice programs must unite with the acute health care system. Spokespersons for the hospice movement, such as Gaetz, Hackley, Lamers, Rezendes, and Saunders, all supported the need for integration with and support from larger institutions. "Donations, special grants, and even out-of-pocket payments do not constitute the stable and reliable types of financing necessary for the support of ongoing service programs. It is important that continuing sources of funding be developed for hospice care" (Osterweis and Champagne 1979, 495).

These advocates applauded policymakers' interest in hospice care and sought out their assistance to teach them ways to break through the health care bureaucracy. Efforts at the community level were largely unsuccessful. Local offices were restricted by regulations, and they did not have the power to create a category for hospice care. Therefore, representatives from hospice programs went to Washington, D.C., to discuss with legislators ways to change regulations to include a hospice benefit. These leaders were not concerned that policymakers would attempt to alter the spirit of the hospice ideal; rather, they asserted that the movement needed to take advantage of the existing popular support for hospice care before public attention turned elsewhere.

Finally, optimists believed that popular interest in hospice care was a sign of changing cultural values toward dying, and they were unconcerned about the potential dangers of integrating with the medical system. "The meteoric increase in hospice care signals a welcome reversal of long-held traditional attitudes denying death and burgeoning acceptance of the compassionate concepts of hospice. In my 23 years in the field I have never seen any one idea catch on as well and as quickly as hospice" (Hackley, quoted in National Conference on Social Welfare 1978, 2).

Rezendes claimed:

> Public consciousness is ready for hospice now. President Carter has called for "effective and low-cost treatment methods" in medicine, avoiding the "duplication of expensive and underutilized equipment and services" and he has urged insurance companies to "write coverage in such a way that it does not stimulate the use of expensive medical procedures and hospital care when less expensive care will be responsive to patients' needs." Hospices provide exactly this sort of program. (Stoddard 1978, 129)

## Impediments to Program Expansion

Many cultural conditions favored the development of hospice programs, but three trends inhibited their expansion: the funding limits placed on creating new institutions, physician disapproval, and cultural concerns that hospice care was another form of euthanasia. At the time hospice care became popular, policymakers favored deinstitutionalization and reduced inpatient bed capacities. Separate facilities, such as Hospice, Inc., or Riverside Hospice, were unpopular. The majority of physicians viewed hospices as a form of hand holding and hospice advocates as pious eccentrics (Butler 1979); they did not accept assertions that hospice care was a continuation of medical treatment. Finally, the value Americans placed on technology aroused concern that hospice philosophy would encourage a precipitous cessation of treatment.

**Funding Limitations** Although many programs developed because of people's enthusiasm and willingness to provide free services, such zeal was not enough. Acquiring funds to start new programs became a continuing quest for early developers. Amenta (1984) reported that by 1980 directors were devoting more time to fund-raising than to providing care.

Most of the individuals who created hospice programs came from the health care system, and medical insurance was the most familiar source of reliable funding. Rezendes reported that in 1975 when Hospice, Inc., was seeking funds, insurers were forthright with him that the best way to make hospice care appealing was to show that it reduced costs. As this knowledge spread, providers asserted that hospice had cost-saving potential to make themselves eligible for insurance reimbursement, despite limited information on the actual costs of hospice care (GAO 1979). Josefina Magno, for example, convinced Blue Cross/Blue Shield that hospice care would reduce patient care costs by 25 percent and then found a Washington, D.C., nursing home to institute a pilot hospice program (Ewens and Herrington 1983).

The easiest access to reimbursement was through billing for home health care services. Hospice care, despite the specialty components of its service, performed tasks that were similar to home health care. The list of billable services included skilled nursing, physical therapy, occupational therapy, social work, and home health assistance. By 1983 the majority of programs (57 percent) provided home health services (McCann 1985).

**Physician Disapproval** Physician resistance was considered a greater threat to the movement's progress. "Major medical research centers have not, for the most part, taken a pioneering or even leading role in developing American hospices" (Ewens and Herrington 1983, 228). Physicians saw hospice staff as morbid do-gooders, and they asserted that hospice care providers were so preoccupied with helping patients die that they forgot to help them live.

Overall providers found themselves trying to garner support for hospice services from physicians who suspected that hospice care represented "giving up" on their patients. As one group explained, during their early years they went to the medical community with their "dog and pony show" to convince physicians that hospice care was credible medical care. Some programs required that the primary physician agree to a hospice program; patient and family could not independently request hospice care. Moreover, the physician determined treatment, and the hospice team did not discuss a patient's terminal status if the patient's physician forbade it. Despite these changes, the majority of physicians did not refer patients, and those that did referred patients so close to death that little could be done to comfort them (Corless 1985).

Physicians did, however, begin to take an interest in pain management techniques. In 1979 the National Institutes of Health sponsored a two-day symposium on the management of pain. Physicians were among the participants. Treatment of all chronic pain was beginning to be a specialty practice, and recognition by medical researchers that new treatments could moderate chronic pain attracted physicians' attention. As a medical specialty, however, pain management became an entity separate from hospice care, and it did not improve physicians' attitudes toward the movement.

**Fear of Euthanasia** Critics of the hospice movement also stated that ceasing aggressive life-saving therapy as prescribed by hospice providers was a form of mercy killing (Rossman 1977). Cohen (1979) asserted that hospice providers must publicize the differences between hospice care and euthanasia so prolife factions would not oppose hospice care. (Cohen's warning was warranted. During the 1980s prolife proponents began to influence abortion laws and individual pleas to cease life-support systems. As a political force, prolife has become a powerful opponent of prochoice and euthanasia proponents. Had hospice advocates not begun early in the movement's history to counter any association with mercy killing, program growth might have been severely restricted by prolife groups.) Hospice providers heeded such warnings and censored attempts to associate hospice with passive euthanasia. As one program representative told me when I interviewed her: "Our publications are copyrighted. You're welcome to use information about our program for your professional writings. However, we will not approve writings that associate our work with euthanasia. One man sent us his manuscript, and we had to refuse him copyright permission because he associated hospice with euthanasia. Euthanasia is the antithesis of hospice."

The National Hospice Organization's committee on bioethics characterized *euthanasia* as an inflammatory word. The committee believed that any association with euthanasia might be picked up by opponents as evidence that hospice care was a form of euthanasia. After some debate, the committee determined not to include it in its statement on hospice ethics.

## Changing Themes in the Provision of Hospice Care

Different program types had different ways of providing services, and over time the original components of care altered as innovations were introduced. Changes occurred in eligibility requirements for admission to hospice programs and in the way that bereavement, pastoral care, and volunteer services were provided. Moreover, the constant effort to obtain funds and attract patient referrals resulted in alterations that made hospice programs more consistent with the traditional medical community.

**Admission Procedures** Programs that admitted all terminally ill patients ultimately found this policy to be impractical. When elderly patients lived alone, with no nearby family or friends to support them, they required excessive staff support. As a result, the personal care provider requirement was established and became a common practice among hospice providers. This criterion meant that to be eligible for services patients had to have at least one person who lived with them, or near them, who would be willing to assume responsibility for their care.

Although volunteers and staff were attracted to hospice care because of their interest in death and dying, such interest did not qualify them to be hospice caregivers; volunteers and staff, inadequately trained, often made up the majority of staff helping families and patients manage death's emotional and physical trauma (Klagsbrun 1982). Lack of training affected the way that caregivers interpreted hospice principles. As hospice programs integrated with health care facilities, the team became less committed to helping patients and families talk about their experiences; instead they concentrated their attention on physical care needs. Providers rationalized their behavior, stating that they took cues from patients; if patients wanted to talk about death, they would do so, but staff did not initiate such discussions. (Curiously, this attitude contradicts research by Feifel [1959], Kübler-Ross [1969], and Glaser and Strauss [1967], which found that it was caregivers' reluctance to talk about death that inhibited patients from asking questions.)

**Counseling Services** Another perversion of hospice services was a consequence of providers who saw communication about death as another treatment process. Caregivers who strictly adhered to Kübler-Ross's stage theory made it "a form of orthodoxy in the hospice context" (Hare 1983, 10), a process each person must traverse with the goal of achieving happy death, rather than a way to encourage communication and normalize the experience. Such providers and families interpreted Kübler-Ross's theory as a blueprint; staff educated families regarding the stages of dying, and families complied by reciting the ways that they traversed the stages, sometimes taking only a weekend to do so. At times those who embraced the theory in this way forgot the individual who was the recipient of their care.

Spiritual and bereavement services, which were unique to hospice care, were not given equal importance by all hospice care providers. Davidson (1978) purported that it was pastoral care that separated hospice services from traditional medical care and that it thus should have been emphasized by providers, but newer programs neither understood nor incorporated spiritual care in their design (Mount 1985; Klagsbrun 1982).

Consistent with medical professionals' tendency to avoid talking about feelings, bereavement counseling never received the attention bestowed on other aspects of hospice care. When the IWG published assumptions and principles regarding hospice care in 1979, Parkes pointed out that the area of bereavement was neglected (Foster 1979). Research on bereavement was also limited (Mount 1985). Contributing to this problem was a lack of reimbursement for bereavement services; as providers integrated with medical care systems their services were shaped by available funding sources. Bereavement counseling was not reimbursed by insurers. Providers therefore stated that although they agreed that this service was important, they could not provide it until monies were found to pay for staff time. Some providers believed that bereavement counseling imposed excessive demands on staff time. Hospice of Marin was among the programs that identified this problem. Ironically, the founder of Hospice of Marin, Lamers, started out to create a center for grief reactions. A year after Hospice of Marin began providing services the staff found that bereavement counseling needs were greater than the staff could manage and consequently limited bereavement services to monthly family meetings (Lamers 1978).

Other programs never even tried to attend to grieving families' counseling needs. They restricted their bereavement services by eliminating counseling services and maintaining contact with survivors through phone calls and condolence cards. A survey of hospice programs found that bereavement was an aspect of hospice service that most providers hoped to be able to upgrade, when funding permitted, from phone calls and condolence cards to site visits following patient death. Families that needed counseling were referred to other agencies (GAO 1979).

Although funding was the biggest impediment to providing bereavement services, provider values also influenced the provision of such services. Programs such as Hospice, Inc., the Brooklyn Hospice, and Kaiser Permanente did not receive reimbursement for counseling, but they still provided a full range of bereavement services, including groups, individual counseling, education, and home visits.

**Staff Interactions with Patients and Families** Another way that hospice care changed as it became part of the medical environment was by encouraging hospice providers to treat patients as objects of care, not as participants, thus forgetting their goal to return control of treatment to patient and family (Mudd 1982). Staff decided on solutions for families, "a deluge of services resulting from a careless assessment may relieve a crisis atmosphere, but it can also produce a quiet sense of helplessness and depression in a family stripped of its responsibility and need to care for its own (13–14)." Staff found themselves doing for patients and families rather than helping them to do for themselves.

Limited funding for hospital-based hospice programs affected service delivery and further evidenced the way that medicalization subsumed efforts to normalize death. Hospice care was initially designed to make staff members available when the patient and family needed them, rather than at the staff's convenience. This meant that staff might visit a family at night because the patient had become acutely ill and the family requested the team's assistance. Hospital-based programs, by contrast, often could not pay staff to be available 24 hours a day, and often operated 9 A.M. to 5 P.M., five or six days a week. Emergency services might be available over the phone, or patient and family were instructed to call hospice emergency services. Consistent with a medicalization process, emphasizing access to medical technology frequently became staff's greatest responsibility, despite the fact that dying was to be a natural, not a medical, event.

Some hospice programs that integrated with traditional health care systems were not able to use volunteers to provide direct services. Insurance coverage, for example, restricted the use of volunteers. In California professionals such as physicians or counselors who wanted to volunteer their services were not covered by malpractice insurance. In New York, acute care hospitals did not allow volunteers to perform personal care. Instead they were assigned traditional tasks, such as bringing patients water or assisting with office work.

**Medical Treatment versus Patient Choice: A Case Study** Ideally, the hospice choice represented the patient's decision to cease curative treatments. As hospice care merged with traditional health care, patients were more likely to have fewer options. Ceasing aggressive treatment and empowering patient and family to make informed decisions were not universal to hospice programs; within hospital-based hospice programs, the distinction between comfort and cure blurred.

> Physicians desiring not to "abandon" their patients often use chemothera-peutic drugs and extensive laboratory services literally until the patient's last breath. The quality of life achieved under these circumstances is often miserable. The physicians do this in the belief that they may help the patient and, if not that person, others in the future. These physicians are not "awful" men and women. They are faced with the dilemma of how to practice medicine with a credo that demands faithfulness to the preservation of human life. (Corless 1983, 341)

The following case description depicts the conflict that resulted from combining hospice care with acute health care. As hospice programs integrated with traditional health care systems, they began to reflect the values of the latter.

Anna was a middle-aged woman suffering from abdominal cancer. For a time she received chemotherapy, which deterred the spread of the disease, but eventually treatments ceased to be effective and Anna was referred to a hospice program. This program was part of an acute health care system that did not require patients to give up aggressive treatments.

Ideally, under these circumstances, the team would have educated Anna about treatment options and encouraged her to decide what to do, but this program deferred to the physician to explain medical options. The physician asserted that chemotherapy benefitted Anna psychologically because it gave her hope that she would get better. Anna did not like the side effects of chemotherapy, but like many patients she was afraid to contradict her physician. The hospice team spoke for her to the physican, who, while sympathetic to Anna's discomfort, opted to continue treatment.

**Hospice Care: How Did It Help?** To balance this discussion of the compromises occurring in hospice care, the following case depicts the way hospice programs were able to improve services for the dying. Participation in the acute health care system was not always negative. The way the hospice team interpreted its role and the way that patients used the services also influenced outcomes. Although the trend in programs was to require a personal care provider, not all programs believed this was necessary. By being less restrictive about who they served, hospice providers often filled a gap in the health care delivery system, as in the following case.

At times hospice providers were able to facilitate patient control over the process, particularly when the physician supported the patient's decisions. Jim was a Vietnam veteran, a loner, who lived in a boardinghouse and suffered from throat cancer. He was aware of the probable course of his disease, suffocation because of tumor pressure on his windpipe. He was frightened by this, discussed it with the hospice physician and decided he wanted to continue treatments, radiation or chemotherapy, to inhibit tumor growth.

Whatever family Jim had were not available to assist him as his illness progressed, and he preferred to keep his own counsel. Attempts by hospice staff to provide emotional support were met with hostile responses from Jim, which were interpreted by staff as his way of saying that he did not want to talk about his feelings. They respected his wishes and focused instead on his physical needs. At the clinic where Jim received his treatments, the hospice nurse met him and checked to make sure that he had a supply of liquid food and that he was able to manage without in-home assistance. One week Jim did not show up for his scheduled appointment. The home care nurse tried to contact Jim's boardinghouse. Failing this, the team decided to wait and see if he would keep the next appointment; when he did not, a home visit was made to see if he needed help.

The team member who visited Jim found that his condition had worsened; he could neither feed himself nor move about his room. He did not want to go to the hospital for more treatment, and his physician concurred. The hospice team helped him to manage at home by hiring a homemaker to assist him with dressing, bathing, and housecleaning. Contrary to his earlier reluctance, he welcomed the team's visits, and the team did their best to ease his anxiety until his death several weeks later.

## Evaluating Hospice Care

The first evaluations of hospice care in this country were predominantly anecdotal accounts or single-case studies of programs' accomplishments. Leaders repeatedly asserted the need for empirical data about hospice care. Research on the distinctions among forms of care, the consequences of the movement's erratic growth, the difference between hospice and nonhospice care, and the benefits of bereavement counseling were minimal. The following is an overview of research on hospice care during the late 1970s and early 1980s, the movement's peak years.

Anecdotal reports depicting hospice benefits made up the bulk of the literature. For example, a nurse in Pennsylvania who used hospice concepts to improve terminally ill patients' quality of life described her experience with 12 patients. As advocate and listener she assisted these patients in negotiating hospital restrictions and achieving more comfort, such as allowing a male patient to wear trousers rather than a hospital gown or teaching a patient's spouse to administer morphine injections, thus allowing the patient to return home. Going home improved this particular patient's condition so much that she was able to cease taking pain medication (Rossman 1977).

Various assessments, not backed up by empirical data, asserted that the hospice movement had created an alternative to the acute health care system. Millett (1979) described hospices as "challenging society's approach to death." According to this author, the hospice movement brought attention to the limited medical research on pain control and patients' preference to die at home. Furthermore, hospices provided social support for families.

> Staff members assess how the family operates in normal circumstances as well as in times of stress. An understanding of the family's coping abilities, decision-making processes, strengths and weaknesses, and areas of tension and conflict, and a knowledge of the role of the patient within the family provides essential information needed by team members to plan appropriate help for the months ahead. The success of home care is dependent in large

part on the active participation of the family in providing physical care as well as emotional support. (Millett 1979, 142–43)

Hospice, Inc., in keeping with its status as the first American hospice, was also the first to empirically study program benefits. Comparing two groups, one receiving hospice care and a control group that did not, researchers found that hospice patients and their primary caregivers experienced significantly less depression, hostility, somaticization (expression of emotional distress through physical complaints), frustration, and dependence than did the nonhospice group (Lack and Buckingham 1978).

The National Hospice Organization also collected data about hospice care; it gathered numbers on patients served, program types, and cost-saving benefits of hospice services. In one 1979 study, NHO assessed the factors that influenced the provision of services. This last project found that the location of the administrative unit determined the method of service delivery. Stated differently, programs administered by an independent staff were more likely to emphasize a pure model of hospice care, whereas programs whose administrative staff had ties to a larger institution would be more likely to allow external demands to influence provision of care.

Comparisons of who hospice providers served and what services they provided showed a pattern; programs tended to represent either medicalized or demedicalized philosophies. Buckingham and Lupu (1982) found that hospice service could be categorized into two types: (1) independent hospice programs that relied on volunteer staff, emphasized psychosocial support of patient and family, and had difficulty surviving financially and (2) institutionally based, professionally staffed programs that emphasized medical treatments, experienced fewer financial problems, and had greater survival rates. Russell's (1985) research repeated these findings and added that independent programs emphasized hospice care as an alternative to acute health care services, while institutional programs emphasized hospice as an extension of these services.

As access to Medicare became a reality, researchers noted that traditional health care reimbursement structures were endangering hospice programs (Connor and Kraymer 1982; Creek 1982; Dooley 1982; Lynn 1985; Mudd 1982). Lack and Buckingham (1978) suggested it would be difficult to traverse the maze of the traditional health care system without changing the purpose and nature of hospice care. Creek (1982) reported that hospice providers found themselves being used by hospitals to expedite discharge for difficult patients. Dooley (1982) pointed out that traditional reimbursement mechanisms were antithetical to hospice philosophy and that hospitals would take staff away from hospice work in times of financial strain.

## A Legitimate Health Care Alternative

In 1982 hospice care providers received financial support from state and federal agencies for hospices services; Medicare, Blue Cross/Blue Shield, and other insurers included hospice services among their benefits. Legitimization meant that hospice programs were licensed alternative health care services, but reimbursement emphasized physical care.

**The Medicare Benefit**  In September 1982 the Tax Equity and Fiscal Responsibility Act (TEFRA) expanded Medicare benefits to create a new hospice benefit. A sunset clause made this benefit temporary. An evaluation of hospice care, completed in September 1986, determined that this benefit should be permanent. The Medicare benefit increased services to terminally ill patients, but it also reflected the medicalizing forces that had dominated the movement's political process. Reimbursement was for physical care services that were consistent with traditional health care's philosophy; other aspects of hospice care, such as spiritual and bereavement support, were not covered.

Briefly stated, policymakers supported the hospice philosophy, but they only reimbursed certain services. The original components of care—an interdisciplinary team, patient participation in treatment decision, pain management and symptom control, and patient and family as the unit of care—were all components of the Medicare hospice benefit.

The hospice benefit was an improvement in services to the terminally ill in several ways. The regulations emphasized home care services and expanded coverage to include assistance to chronically ill patients. Moreover, the Medicare regulations required hospice programs to have team members who were trained specialists and worked directly for the hospice program. Programs had to have as staff members—paid or volunteer—nurses, social workers, medical directors, and counseling personnel.

Patients had the choice of opting for the hospice benefit, which supported the idea that patients should control treatments. They did not have to be acutely ill to qualify for services, nor were they disqualified from receiving services because their condition stabilized. Thus, patients received daily assistance from homemakers or home health aides, and nurses, too, could visit daily to provide physical care or psychosocial support. Counseling services for families and patients were also mandated services. Furthermore, when a patient became a recipient of hospice services, it was the hospice team who had final say over the patient's medical care, not the personal physician.

The Medicare benefit, however, fell far short of hospice providers' expectations, particularly in regard to reimbursement for hospice services. Initially, those who disagreed with the regulations did what the government invited them to do—they responded to the various stipulations regarding coverage. Their negative responses focused on four issues: the cap placed on reimbursement, the restrictions on inpatient services, the expectation that patients must acknowledge their terminal status, and the lack of reimbursement for bereavement and spiritual services.

First, the Medicare regulations restricted the amount of money to cover patient services. With some adjustment to account for differences in area costs, the total reimbursement for a patient receiving hospice services during a six-month period would be $6,500. Although legislators agreed that hospice providers should provide extensive supportive services, the reimbursement rate reflected an expectation that family and volunteers would provide the bulk of physical care. Moreover, death at home became a mandate, not a patient choice; Medicare rules restricted acute inpatient stays to 20 percent of the total length of stay and respite care to a five-day period, thus forcing hospice providers to fulfill their assertions that patients wanted to die at home.

Another controversial Medicare regulation was that patients had to agree to having hospice services. This raised concern among some providers that patients were being forced to acknowledge their terminal status. Programs had always vacillated in their appreciation of Kübler-Ross's theory on patients' desire to talk about death. These providers asserted that patients would discuss their death if they wanted to; they did not believe in forcing patients to do so or in requiring them to sign an agreement indicating their willingness to give up curative treatments to be eligible for hospice benefits.

Finally, the proposed benefits did not reimburse for bereavement and pastoral care services. The Medicare regulations did affirm that bereavement services were a necessary component of hospice care, but they did not reimburse them. Perhaps the greatest irony was Medicare's stipulations regarding spiritual support. The hospice concept owed much to the religious men and women who found the resources and built up the political support needed to develop early programs. Often volunteer programs existed because clergy, who believed in the importance of humane care for the dying, donated their time to coordinate the programs. Not only did the regulations deny funding for pastoral care, they specified that nurses, volunteers, or other team members could provide spiritual supports.

**Adjustments in the Medicare Benefit**   The first change in the regulations occurred in 1984 to accommodate rural hospice programs' special needs. Programs in rural areas that started providing services before 1983 were allowed to call themselves hospices even if their only full-time staff was a nurse coordinator. Moreover, these providers could request exemption from the Medicare regulation that required them to contract directly for services. This last ruling was made because independent rural programs with small caseloads could not support salaries for a separate staff.

In 1985 the Consolidated Omnibus Budget Reconciliation Act (COBRA) made hospice care a permanent part of the Medicare program. Up to that time, expenditures for hospice care totaled $71 million, a far cry from the predicted $160 billion. Furthermore, COBRA raised the hospice benefit and permitted states to provide hospice services under the Medicaid program (Tames 1986).

The final amendment to the Medicare regulations occurred in 1989 when the per patient cap was raised to $9,010, but the daily reimbursement rate remained fixed regardless of level of care needed, and it favored home care services. Federal fears that hospice care would drain Medicare funds rather than save them persisted even though research sponsored by the government found that home care hospice programs could reduce costs. Moreover, those familiar with this data suggested that legislators' analyses of hospice costs were questionable (Corless 1985).

The restrictions imposed on hospice services by Medicare were typical of the Reagan administration. The federal government funded little; monies were to be obtained from state and local funds. Thus Medicare coverage was limited to physical care, such as nursing services; other aspects of hospice care were to be paid by other sources.

"TEFRA was better known as the legislation that raised taxes by almost $100 billion over the ensuing three years and cut social programs sharply. Medicare spending over the three-year period was cut by $13 billion" (Hoyer 1990, 30).[3] Hospice care was included in the TEFRA legislation because hospice leaders were relentless in lobbying for its inclusion and because legislators and the administration saw it as a way to offer a new service while they reduced Medicare spending (Keller and Bell 1984). They were not pro-hospice, but pro-cost reduction.

**JCAH and Insurers Approve Hospice Services** Concurrent with the establishment of a Medicare hospice benefit, the Joint Commission on Accreditation of Hospitals (JCAH) established standards for hospice care. The JCAH standards did not favor one organizational model or stipulate patient length of stay, but they required a full complement of hospice services for program accreditation. These standards particularly affected hospital-based programs. Failure to conform with JCAH hospice standards meant that the hospital's accreditation would be revoked. Hospice programs in hospitals that provided a case management approach to terminal care with perhaps one nurse as the program's staff had to expand the program or call themselves by another name if they did not want to lose their JCAH accreditation.

Other insurers accepted hospice care as an alternative consumer choice, but they restricted coverage in ways that were similar to the Medicare program. For example, Equitable covered a lifetime maximum of $5,000, of which $300 was allocated for bereavement services. Metropolitan Life had a $7,000 cap for room and board, allowed seven days for respite care, and reimbursed selectively for bereavement services that enhanced the patient's and the family's peace of mind. Hartford Life was the most generous in that it placed no reimbursement limits on physical care, but did restrict social work services to $100 before death and $100 after death (NHO 1985). (It will not surprise the reader to note that Hartford Life, a Connecticut-based insurer, was more generous in its reimbursement. Its provider, Hospice, Inc., was generally more successful than other hospice programs in obtaining funding.)

## Conclusion

As hospice programs became popular and became integrated with the health care system, those aspects of hospice services that were not consistent with traditional health care's values were downplayed or ignored. The rhetoric of the movement suggested that attention to spiritual care and bereavement services was important, but neither was a priority in service provision. Rather, providers asserted that bereavement and spiritual services would be improved once they obtained reimbursement for these services.

By the end of this peak period of the hospice movement, the form that hospice programs took was a result of the funding available rather than the movement's ideals. The value conflict inherent to the movement's ideals—normalizing death versus treating death's pains—was never articulated by core members, and no attempt was made to address the inconsistencies that these values created in the movement's goals. Politically the movement directed its efforts toward gaining access to reimbursement from the health care industry. This also influenced programs in that they emphasized physical care needs—the services that were covered under existing health care insurance.

The dominant factor that explains the alteration in program goals was not that policymakers or medical entrepreneurs subsumed reform efforts. They simply took advantage of an opportunity presented to them by hospice providers. Rather, it was the tolerance that hospice leaders had for medical settings and practices that co-opted the hospice movement. Core leaders did not argue strongly against integrating hospice services with health care systems; most applauded this idea as the optimum way to increase the number of programs. Integration with the medical system brought hospice care to the attention of medical entrepreneurs who subsequently joined the movement. These new participants might have some interest in helping the dying, but they also were interested in insurance reimbursement and expanding health care services.

Those participants who believed that reforming medical care had to be accomplished from without, not from within, conformed to, or were overshadowed by, other leaders. Community-oriented programs with small, primarily volunteer staff had greater difficulty surviving, and they did not shape the political course of the movement.

*Chapter 7*

# Fragmentation

In September 1982 providers of hospice care became eligible for reimbursement under the Medicare program. Some movement leaders questioned the legislation. Would it facilitate or impede their cause? Providers had assumed that the Medicare benefit would provide adequate reimbursement for all hospice services and all program types; in reality it restricted funds to services that were congruent with traditional medical care and favored the home care model. Fragmentation occurred as leaders and providers who had been unified during the process of applying for reimbursement became divided once the Medicare legislation had passed.

Idealists who had developed the first hospice programs avowed that these regulations inhibited the creative and humanistic qualities of hospice care and forced one program type—the home care model—on all providers rather than allowing program type to be dictated by community need. Medical entrepreneurs and policy analysts asserted that the Medicare regulations stabilized program quality and made hospice care a credible health service. They favored participation with the Medicare program as a way to expand what was characterized as the "hospice industry." Most hospice providers were against participating because the program did not reimburse services adequately.

Although providers blamed the Medicare regulations for their problems, research showed that the movement had failed to produce an alternative service for the dying (Seale 1989). Hospice care had become a part of the "medical industrial complex" (Relman 1987). Certain original ideals, such as normalizing grief, were inadequately supported by the majority of hospice providers.

Regardless of program structure, the concept of hospice care did have its benefits. Although hospice care was ineffective in alleviating of all death's pains, it created a supportive work environment for health care professionals and reduced family stress. Moreover, hospice care tempered medical treatment for the dying; patients who opted for this service were less likely to be subjected to unnecessary tests and aggressive treatments during the last days of life.

For a time the hospice "industry" flourished, but the movement's ability to reform medical care for the dying diminished. New providers emerged who complied with the Medicare regulations, some older programs adapted to conform to the requirements of Medicare funding, and the first for-profit hospice chain was created. By the late 1980s, programs languished from lack of referrals and inadequate reimbursement rates. Institutionally affiliated program growth stagnated, and many providers struggled for fiscal survival; limited access to insurance dollars led to program failure as health care costs rose, private sources of support were directed to more pressing social problems, and financially strapped medical systems shrugged off programs that were not income producing.

All of the above developments are expected in the fourth stage of a social movement's development—fragmentation—according to stage theory. Stage theory recognizes that the achievements of the third phase—institutionalization—come at a price. Co-optations and deflections are recognized by movement leaders. Some accept the changes that have occurred, while others oppose them. Disagreement and friction between idealists and newer recruits is common; original leaders are characterized as unrealistic fanatics and are pushed out of the movement's political process. Concomitantly, participants begin to withdraw, believing that conditions have improved. The hospice movement departed from this course in that leaders who opposed the changes were not easily pushed aside and that many idealists remained active providers of hospice care. Therefore, rather than proceeding quickly from the stage of fragmentation to demise, the movement was kept alive by participants who continued to try to reform terminal care.

## The Disruptive Effect of Medicare Legislation

Politically, the movement continued to emphasize access to reimbursement rather than provision of hospice services. Although united in their belief that public funding would benefit the hospice industry, leaders were divided in their views of the new reimbursement program. Publication of the Medicare regulations created widespread controversy among hospice participants; for the first time in-house debates erupted. Many providers were outraged at the limitations that the Medicare regulations placed on services, while others claimed that hospice participants needed to be realistic in their expectations.

At first disputes among participants were tempered by providers' belief that the proposed regulations would not go into effect in their original form. As it turned out, the regulations not only preserved their original intent but further reduced the reimbursement rate. "When HCFA [Health Care Financing Administration] published the final rules in December 1983 it lowered home care reimbursement to $46.25, down from $53.17 per day" (Tames 1986, 3). Philosophical and political differences that had heretofore peacefully coexisted erupted as leaders and participants fought over the Medicare legislation.

> A major squabble erupted within the hospice movement. The riff [*sic*] took the form of philosophical division between two factions; those that favored the federally reimbursed, hospice care concept and those that felt that to achieve true hospice care, volunteer staffed hospice should be accountable only to the patient and family. Some hospice supporters felt hospice should not only deal with emotional and spiritual needs of the patient and family, but the disease related medical needs as well, which realistically meant accepting reimbursement. (Williams 1989, 15)

Those who supported the Medicare legislation characterized it as a success because hospice care had become a legitimate alternative to the acute health care system (Gray-Toft and Anderson 1983; Paradis 1988). Medicare reimbursement stabilized the industry and gave programs clear guidelines for providing services; now that the Medicare regulations were established, providers could go ahead with the task of making hospice services available nationally.

Medical entrepreneurs also saw the Medicare benefit as a boost to the hospice industry. This group viewed hospice care as a business and had a hard time understanding what all the fuss was about. They believed that hospice programs should adapt to current reimbursement structures and provide services within these constraints. The theme of an NHO meeting reflects this position: "Melding Ideals with Reality."

Many leaders, who had entered the movement during the institutional stage, were sympathetic to the acute health care system. They agreed that

health care should be rationally managed (i.e., providing quality care, effi-
ciently and cost-effectively) and that nonmedical treatments should not be
functions of hospice programs. For example, admitting a dying person for
inpatient care to reduce the family's emotional and physical stress was
fiscally irresponsible, and Medicare regulations made hospice providers
more responsible (Tehan 1985).

> The practice of hospice care is dramatically different than it was ten years
> ago. This change, by itself, is not necessarily bad. Ten years ago there was
> no accepted standard of practice, no utilization review, and only token
> attempts to contain costs. If the patient was dying at home and the family
> wanted their relative hospitalized, the hospice staff would readily facilitate
> the transfer. Today, the nurse in a Medicare certified hospice must assess
> whether the patient's condition warrants the skilled intervention of an acute
> care hospital. Just because a person is dying is no justification for an in-
> patient admission. (Tehan 1985, 11–12)

Purists, viewed as unrealistic idealists, wanted to maintain the original
spirit of hospice care.

> Hospice work is lonely, hard, and frightening. It does not always engender
> gratefulness, and it frequently causes depression for everyone concerned.
> This work cannot be done alone; it is complicated. A community-based
> hospice that offers consultative help to families, physicians, or nurses must
> have actual hospital beds built into the system. These beds must be available
> at will to function as a part of the hospice or to function in a hospice light.
> Hospice work therefore requires cooperative effort that includes total care
> from hospital to home. A group of people who can take care of each other
> while they are taking care of dying patients and their families is needed.
> And with this community of people, a financial base is needed. (Klagsbrun
> 1983, 25)

Idealists believed that the Medicare benefit impaired hospice providers'
ability to provide a full complement of hospice services. "Having settled
for half a loaf as the best that could be obtained at the present time, the
leaders of the hospice movement may have made a serious miscalculation.
The half loaf may simply be crumbs unable to give succor to the needs of
the vast array of individuals with far advanced disease" (Corless 1985,
296). Idealists also believed that participants should reject the idea of
tying hospice care to reimbursement strategies: hospices should not be in

the business of competing for health care dollars, and dying should not be viewed solely as a medical problem (Lynn 1985).

Providers, who wanted Medicare benefits but were disappointed with its restrictions, asserted that NHO had sold out hospice ideals. Suspicion that the membership had been duped was supported by participants in the demonstration project. As Greer, the chief investigator of the HCFA-commissioned National Hospice Study, stated, "While the evaluators were amusing themselves testing their hypotheses objectively, the special interests maintained their unrelenting pressure on Congress. The result was the inclusion of hospice in the Medicare reimbursement system before completion of the National Hospice Study" (Greer 1985, 84).

The majority of participants fought the proposed regulations; they wanted more money and legislative support of different program types. Hospice professionals were independent thinkers and self-starters who did not easily conform to bureaucratic structures. As news of the Medicare regulations reached them, independent thinking prevailed, and they refused to apply for Medicare benefits. As mentioned earlier, three programs were approved; 26 were pending approval during 1983, the first year that the regulations went into effect. By 1986, when hospice became a permanent benefit of the Medicare program, there were only 275 certified programs (Tames 1986). By 1988 only 531 out of a possible 1,500 programs were approved (Jones 1988).

A new study by the U.S. Government Accounting Office (1989) assessed provider resistance to Medicare and found the following: providers were opposed to six-month life expectancy for hospice patients; they were unable to comply with the expectation that hospice programs have their own physicians, nurses, social workers, and counselors; and they opposed the cap for total cost of services.

## Benefits and Restrictions:
## Hospice Services in the 1980s

By the time Medicare regulations were enacted the most common form of hospice program was the community-based home care program. Such programs benefitted families, explaining the disease process and helping to make the patient comfortable. Home care programs also had drawbacks. They did not always have access to funds or to volunteers to meet the day-to-day home care needs of patients, and their services were predominantly nursing oriented. The following case is indicative of the movement's achievements; hospice care represented more than had existed before, but it fell short of meeting all of the movement's goals.

Mrs. R. was an educated, white, middle-class woman in her early 60s suffering from breast cancer who had a supportive family. For two years after her initial diagnosis Mrs. R. received chemotherapy to prevent further spread of her disease. When treatments failed to achieve their desired results and Mrs. R.'s condition weakened, she opted to cease treatment and agreed to be referred to a hospice program for supportive services.

The first interaction Mrs. R. and her family had with the hospice team was in regard to Mrs. R.'s physical discomfort. Mrs. R.'s physician, now that she had been deemed untreatable, was less available for consultation and Mrs. R. was often in pain. The hospice nurse and social worker discussed the situation with Mrs. R. and her family. They suggested that the physician might not be comfortable managing this phase of the illness and that there were other physicians who worked well with terminally ill patients. Mrs. R. agreed to switch doctors and the hospice staff, in conjunction with the new physician, were able to alleviate her physical discomfort. The hospice team continued to keep Mrs. R. pain-free for the remainder of her life; at times she was sluggish or uncomfortable, but she was never in acute distress.

As the disease progressed Mrs. R. weakened physically. Her family did not live with her, and they requested in-home assistance. This hospice program was freestanding; it did not have an inpatient service and did not have volunteers to compensate for expensive homemaker services. Mrs. R.'s benefits provided only for part-time home care services, and she did not have a great deal of financial resources to supplement her health care benefits. Therefore her family had to take care of her. During the latter stages of her illness they took turns staying overnight at their mother's home.

Eventually, Mrs. R. became so weak and the family so exhausted from caregiving while maintaining their responsibilities to spouses and jobs that they decided to seek inpatient services. Because Mrs. R. did not require acute health care services she could not be admitted to a hospital. The only other option was a nearby terminal care facility that had some hospice characteristics. This facility provided palliative services, but did not encourage family involvement in patient care decisions.

The family and Mrs. R. assembled and concluded that although they would prefer that Mrs. R. remain at home, this was not possible. They notified the hospice team of their decision and the social worker arranged for Mrs. R.'s admission, which took place a few days later.

The family was displeased with the institutional care their mother received. They felt that after months of caring for her at home they knew what made Mrs. R. feel better. For example, Mrs. R. seemed to perk up when she was able to sit in a wheelchair and go outside with her children, but the facility only got people out of bed at certain times of the day, and these were not times when the family could visit. Feeding was another problem; Mrs. R. had always been a hearty eater but no attempt was made to cater to her appetite. Instead, she was fed pureed foods.

Mrs. R. died soon after her admission to the facility, and the family was left to cope with their grief. The hospice program sent condolence cards, but no team member met with the family to discuss their feelings and no suggestions were made about community groups for grieving family members.

## The Movement Matures

By 1990, 39 states had established licensing for hospice programs, and at least 16 insurers reimbursed for hospice services (Hoyer 1990). Although estimates ranged from 1,200–1,700 programs, NHO put the number of hospice programs at 1,500 in 1985 and 1,450 in 1990. Programs that were approved Medicare providers were predominantly home health hospice programs, located in the South and the Northwest (Kidder 1987).

Annual conferences changed, and there was little intimacy or informal sharing of information about hospice goals. Instead, conferences had become places where administrators and entrepreneurs promoted the medical model and angry providers fought to preserve program integrity. Presentations at meetings also changed. One could still discuss ways to help patient and family manage grief reactions or meet spiritual needs, but a new phrase crept into the rhetoric at these meetings, "how to market hospice." New sessions were offered to help educate providers regarding ways to increase their census.

New organizations developed. Some were created by hospice leaders who were dissatisfied with the National Hospice Organization, and others represented an attempt to clarify hospice services for certain groups. The American Society of Hospice Care, started in Boston, and the Hospice Association of America, started in the Washington, D.C., area, were established to compete with NHO and reassert hospice ideals. The former published the *American Journal of Hospice Care* and held annual conferences regarding hospice care. The latter published the newsletter *Hospice Forum* and supported local conferences. The Hospice Association of America (HAA) also credits its congressional lobbying effort with being responsible for the increase in hospice benefits in 1989. "The rate increase was the primary legislative goal of the HAA in 1989. It was a goal which proved to be very difficult, seemingly elusive, and impossible. It was, however, a goal which was very satisfying when ultimately achieved" (Neigh 1990, 13). The Jewish Hospice Commission, a local organization formed in Los Angeles, integrated concepts of hospice care with Jewish tradition and religious values.

By 1985 Foster and Paradis identified 2,000 publications on hospice-related topics, most of which had been published after 1980. Journals aimed at hospice providers were also created. The *American Journal of Hospice Care*, mentioned above, was first published in 1984. (In 1990 it became the *American Journal of Hospice and Palliative Care*.) This journal published research articles, but it also made readers aware of meetings, legislative changes, new programs, equipment, and new drugs. The *Hospice Journal*, first published in 1985 by NHO, took a different approach. It was not geared to public interest but to empirical research. Another noteworthy publication was the Canadian *Journal of Palliative Care*, first published in 1985. Each of these journals is still published.

There also were new problems for the movement leaders, particularly the AIDS epidemic and the concomitant need for special services. AIDS patients were stigmatized by society, and most traditional caregivers were reluctant to provide services. NHO announced that hospice providers were committed to caring for AIDS patients, but hospice programs that were part of traditional health care systems were reluctant to do so, and they found ways to restrict AIDS patients from admission. For example, a home health agency in New York stated that it could not accept AIDS patients because most continued to receive aggressive treatment and therefore did not fit this program's admission criteria.

**Hospice Programs: Old and New** Periodically the literature hinted that hospice programs were having a harder time surviving (Millett 1979). By the early 1980s the difficulty of creating or sustaining programs became an acknowledged problem (Aiken and Marx 1982; Corless 1983; Enck 1986; Klagsbrun 1982; Simson and Wilson 1986).

Insurers favored hospice home care services, but providers tried to maintain their tradition of idiosyncratic program development based on community needs. "Few programs have beautiful gardens like those at Saint Christopher's . . . But, all hospices do have to emphasize palliation and the care of the whole family. Between these is a large area of uncertainty and corresponding danger that whoever established standards may draw the line too narrowly" (Hare 1983, 10). Holding onto beliefs meant, however, that providers could not support themselves; they sought ways to compensate for threats to the movement's survival.

Some hospice providers adapted to or circumvented the limitations imposed by Medicare. For example, providers adapted to the restrictions placed on inpatient stays by requiring that patients' significant others sign contracts stating that they would maintain the person at home until death. And they circumvented Medicare's stipulation on physician referral by giving patients and families whose physicians did not refer them to hospice programs the names of physicians who favored such services.

Overall, Medicare regulations were a disappointment to those providers who had anticipated full support of hospice programs. Without such reliable financing, programs had difficulty surviving. Medicare reimbursement rates encouraged providers to restrict services to nontreatment-oriented, supportive care. Consequently, patients who might require radiation or surgical procedures for comfort, not cure, might be refused admission to programs.

Providers who had counted on more liberal funding for hospice services from the Medicare benefit had to alter their program design. These providers accessed funding in informal ways or, in some cases, changed their names. Saint Luke's Hospice in New York, the second oldest hospice in the country, became a palliative care unit because it would not accept Medicare regulations. This provider believed that restrictions on inpatient stays and medical interventions were not in the best interest of its patients or in keeping with its philosophy.

Independent hospice programs that were created by the National Cancer Institute's demonstration projects had varying levels of success supporting themselves under the Medicare reimbursement structure. Riverside Hospice in New Jersey and Hillhaven Hospice in Tucson had to close their inpatient facilities because reimbursement was not adequate to support an independent facility. They did not cease to exist, but were forced to merge their programs with nearby hospitals. Riverside Hospice became a component of Riverside Hospital, and Hillhaven Hospice was made part of Saint Mary's Hospital. Kaiser Permanante in Norwalk, California, another demonstration project, was part of a large health maintenance organization, and membership dollars compensated for inadequate

Medicare funding. This program, therefore, survived intact, but the Kaiser Permanente network did not build other independent facilities. Future hospice programs developed by this HMO were home care programs. Programs that came to depend on Medicare reimbursement often operated at a loss. For example, Hospice of Northern Virginia claimed that it lost $1,400 per patient, and an NHO report estimated that the average hospice program would lose $106,518 annually because of inadequate Medicare reimbursement (Tames 1986).

New programs placed greater emphasis "on survival and fiscal accountability and less on individual commitment to the hospice concept" (Tehan 1985, 13). The rise of new programs was attributed to the existence of a prospective payment system rather than providers' belief in the movement's mission. Those aspects of hospice care that had made it attractive to participants during the 1970s were subsumed by a new business-oriented hospice provider. A visitor to a hospice program that was created after the mid-1980s might not realize that the psychological and spiritual needs of the dying and their significant others had once been important aspects of hospice care. New programs resembled traditional medical systems, and psychosocial or spiritual concerns were secondary to treatment protocols. Greer and Mor suggested "the politically oriented legislation results in a program that differs substantially from the [hospice] movement that spawned it" (1985, 6). Researchers labeled this a conservative trend (Abel 1986) or tendency toward homogeneity (Paradis and Cummings 1986).

Service provision in newer programs was based on Medicare stipulations, not on the original components of care. As one program coordinator told me, "If you want to begin a hospice program you have to look to the Medicare regulations for guidance. These regulations tell us the best way to provide quality terminal care." Most new programs were extensions of home health care agencies, and their primary emphasis was on the palliative care of patients and education of families about the patient's illness.

The Brooklyn Hospice altered its services because of Medicare regulations (Liss-Levinson 1983). Originally, this program intended to create a separate 10-bed unit, along with home care intensive nursing and social services as well as other services. Funding restrictions meant that certain services had to be altered or eliminated. Specifically, a separate unit was not financially viable; people who required inpatient services were admitted selectively to a skilled nursing facility, where they received care from the same staff that tended other nursing home patients.

The Ritter-Scheuer Hospice Program, which opened in 1983 shortly after the Medicare law was enacted, was an example of a program that failed because of inadequate use of their services and inadequate reimbursement. This program combined home care with a 16-bed inpatient unit. Administratively, it was a separate service within a large hospital/nursing home facility in New York. When the program was created the hospital's board of directors anticipated a financial deficit, but in 1989, when the deficit reached $506,000, despite insurance reimbursement and fund-raising efforts, the program had to close. Although Medicare planned to raise the total cap on services the following year, it would not have been enough to offset Ritter-Scheuer's financial losses (Sack 1989).

In general, researchers found that different program types experienced diverse problems trying to survive the Medicare reimbursement structure (Greer and Mor 1985). Home health programs fared best, but they were financially strained when patients required acute hospital care. They then turned to nursing homes for inpatient care, but nursing homes were not equipped to provide adequate pain management (Buckingham 1982–83; Lynn 1985). Independent hospices served patients who were self-referred, and such patients were admitted to hospice programs earlier in their illness and used more highly skilled staff. These programs were unable to restrict costs to Medicare caps and had to supplement their operating costs. Finally, hospital-based programs had difficulty meeting the needs of patients living far away from the hospital; once admitted for inpatient care, these patients were harder to discharge. Moreover, the latter programs depended on hospital administration to supplement their costs, and as financially strained institutions needed to reduce costs, they were likely to restrict funding for services that were not self-sustaining.

The newest approach to hospice care was the for-profit hospice chain that sought to increase the number of hospices based on an administrative formula, not community need. Donald Gaetz, former executive member of NHO, was the first to attempt it. Starting with a Miami-based program called Hospice Care, Inc., this service spread, and by 1990 it had programs in Florida, Illinois, Massachusetts, and Texas. These programs emphasized home care services and leased space from hospitals to create "hospice houses," a home-like setting for terminally ill patients who could not be maintained at home.

For-profit programs charged for their services. If insurance companies did not pay, or did not pay adequately, patients and families could purchase services. Fees for nursing, home health, and social services were among the charged services, but in keeping with the low value placed on bereavement and spiritual care, fees for these services were minimal or nonexistent.

Medically affiliated programs were the norm, but volunteer community programs persisted. They were not included in demonstration projects, and they were not reimbursed for their services. These programs continued to offer families psychosocial support in the way that they always had—visiting and talking with patients and families about the dying process and helping families cope with their grief. Their funding was minimal, but their staff were trained professionals who volunteered their services because they believed in facilitating death with dignity.

Amidst these limitations and restrictions on service provision there were exceptions. In West Palm Beach an independent inpatient hospice facility opened in the mid-1980s that was dedicated to AIDS patients. This was one of the first new inpatient facilities that was not a component of a hospital or nursing home to be built since the NCI demonstration project in the late 1970s. Officially, it was categorized as a "special hospital," not a hospice, and it was funded by the Robert Wood Foundation as part of a $17.2 million grant given to 11 cities to create humane, inexpensive treatment for AIDS patients.

**The Affects of Change on Movement Participants**  Newer programs developed according to Medicare stipulations, and nurses took leading roles in their organization and administration. In hospice programs, nurses had assumed positions of preeminence; it was the nurse coordinator who determined policy as well as who received what services. Nurses expanded their role to include tasks normally performed by other professionals. A study of social work services in hospice programs found that nurses were more likely to perform social work functions than social workers (Kulys and Davis 1986). Moreover, it was nurses who typically provided spiritual support (Amenta 1988). The standards for hospice programs designated nurses as program coordinators, and staff nurses were allowed autonomy to make palliative care decisions whereas other team members were supervised by the programs' medical directors.

Participation in hospice programs improved nurses' job satisfaction (Vachon 1986). In hospice programs nurses were older, experienced a greater sense of control over their work (Krekorian and Moser 1985), and were significantly more satisfied with their jobs than were hospital-based nurses who dealt with death and dying. Social workers, however, were not better off. Parry (1983) found that there was no difference between hospice social workers' and other medical social workers' job satisfaction.

Volunteer participation in hospices declined (Carney, Borbst, and Burns 1989). Labierte and Mor (1988) did not find that Medicare influenced the use of volunteers as much as did program type. Freestanding institutions (home health programs not connected to hospitals, nursing homes, or home health agencies) used volunteers more than institutionally based programs. As the majority of programs affiliated with home health agencies, the demographic pattern for volunteers also changed; volunteers were older and their turnover was higher. Volunteers expressed feeling helpless to perform the tasks assigned them and disappointed with the way hospice programs functioned. Specifically, volunteers felt overwhelmed and poorly equipped to help families through bereavement (Seibold, Rossi, Bertotti, Sopriych, McQuillan 1987).

The change in volunteer participation reflects the medicalizing influences on hospice care. Programs were composed primarily of paid staff, and volunteers were not as integral to the patient care process. Moreover, volunteers were to perform those aspects of hospice care not covered by insurance reimbursement. Community members who volunteered their services to hospice programs often did so because they believed in providing humane care for terminally ill people, but they were disappointed with the way that many hospice providers interpreted the philosophy of hospice care. Sheehan (1987) stated that the medicalization of hospice care would yield "a high rate of disillusionment and burnout, and hospice will become equated with unfulfilled promises" (6).

The charismatic leaders of the movement were also less visible. Cicely Saunders no longer visited from England; it was suggested that her husband's health precluded such visits. Elisabeth Kübler-Ross continued to advocate dying patients' needs, particularly those of AIDS patients, but her presence was less visible in the movement's political processes. Other idealists, such as William Lamers and Florence Wald, were no longer involved in the hospice programs they started. Early hospice participants were characterized as naive idealists. Williams (1990) described early zealots' activities as resembling the old Andy Hardy movies where Mickey Rooney, usually aided by Judy Garland, got the kids of the town mobilized to start a show and raise money for a worthy cause. The first groups to start hospice programs, according to Williams, were like enthusiastic kids who had little experience or understanding of reality.

As hospice care became part of the insured health care system, the number of entrepreneurs involved increased. Business executives and hospital administrators became common members of hospice boards, replacing the community representatives who had occupied these positions (Paradis and Cummings 1986).

Dying patients had never been active participants in designing hospice services, and as programs medicalized, their input disappeared. The testimonials from patients that had been so popular during the 1970s were less frequent. New programs might place stories about patients receiving their care in local papers in order to introduce their services. Research assessing patients' satisfaction with hospice services relied on family and caregivers' reports. Patients were not asked what they thought (Hays and Arnold 1986; Wilkinson 1986). The problem with such a strategy is that survivors and caregivers, because of the emotional impact that death has on them, do not accurately assess the dying person's response. They will often misconstrue the response to reflect their own wish that the person's last days have been made easier because of their intervention.

**A Scarcity of Patients** As programs proliferated, problems leaders had thought to be short term became chronic. In particular, the majority of hospice programs did not have sufficient referrals to support their existence. There were a number of reasons for inadequate referrals: physicians' limited use of hospice services, short patient stays, competition with other health care providers, and consumers' limited interest in or knowledge of hospice programs.

Although a number of physicians worked in hospices by the mid-1980s, the movement's leaders still asserted that physicians did not support the concept of hospice care, and research suggested that doctors did not utilize hospice care in the way providers desired. Studies stated that physicians resisted hospice programs because they interfered with the patient/doctor relationship (Kohrman 1985) and because physicians had difficulty acknowledging death (Bulkin and Lukashok 1988). Medical schools did not teach physicians hospice philosophy, and medical students did not learn that cessation of treatment was an acceptable option (Wanzer, Federman, Adelstein, et al. 1989). When physicians did refer patients to hospice programs it was for their support services; they were unwilling to avail themselves of hospice personnel's expertise in managing patient care (Corr and Corr 1983).

Research also suggested that some efforts were being made to change medical education. For example, in an effort to re-educate physicians, a hospice preceptorship program was developed at the University of Pennsylvania (Cassileth, Brown, Lavierte, et al. 1989). The program gave medical students the opportunity to work in a hospice and observe medical practice from a different perspective. These students noted the dehumanizing effects of traditional medical care. "The patient was left naked on the bed and unnoticed while she asked for help, and the patient was not touched or asked how she felt while medical personnel examined wounds and drew blood" (262). These students were also impressed by what they learned of terminal patients needs. "It made me realize that you don't always have miraculous words to heal someone's hurt; you can just be there and try to understand" (263). Such programs remained the exception rather than the rule. Their long-term effects have not been studied.

Medicare regulations did not improve relations between hospice care providers and primary physicians. The regulations asserted that a patient must be informed of his or her terminal status before being referred to a hospice program and that the hospice team's recommendations took precedence over those of the primary physician, thus increasing physician opposition to the hospice concept (Kidder 1987). One study found that the 25 percent of physicians who had large caseloads of terminally ill patients (25 or more patients) did not use hospice programs at all. Those physicians who utilized hospice services did so because their patients and families required the added in-home support (Gochman and Bonham 1988).

Patients admitted to hospice programs were often close to death. Delayed referrals meant that the hospice team would provide physical care for terminally ill patients, but they would not be able to assess or treat patients' and families' emotional and physical distress. "Penwood's [a pseudonym for a hospice in Pennsylvania] doctors lamented the fact that patients waited too long to enter the program: 'Hospice isn't just for dying!' " (Munley 1983, 37).

The majority of patients were referred during the last week of life (Corless 1985), and MacDonald (1989) found that one third of the patients referred to New York hospice programs died before admission. Independent programs typically had longer stays than programs affiliated with other health care services, but very few patients (8.5 percent) exceeded a 210-day stay (Moinpour, Polisar, and Conrad 1990). Medicare regulations further reduced the length of stay; hospice providers were reluctant to admit patients who might require protracted care or inpatient services that would cost more than the allotted per-patient cap (Tenney 1988; Wilkinson, MacDonald, and Pelz 1990). Despite efforts to counteract these trends, delayed referrals persisted. Patients admitted to hospice programs were sicker and the length of stay and number of patients declined (Carney, Borbs, and Burns 1989; Lerman 1988).

Another reason for limited use of hospice programs was the lack of public awareness of or interest in hospice. Research indicated that the public was not unduly displeased with traditional health care services (Sarah Lawrence conference 1984) and that it was reluctant to accept hospice care if that meant giving up access to aggressive treatment (Kidder 1987). Moreover, knowledge about hospice care continued to be limited to better educated, higher-income families (Richman and Rosenfield 1988). One study found that 75 percent of their sample were unaware of hospice services, although after viewing a tape 66 percent reported that they would seek hospice services for themselves (Perolloz and Mollica 1981).

Competition with nursing homes and home care agencies also influenced use of services. Hospice programs were rarely in competition with one another, but frequently competed with area hospitals, nursing homes, and home health agencies for market share (Kidder 1987). Hospice programs developed at a time when the health care industry was struggling financially and various institutions were competing to maintain adequate referrals. As another health care option, hospice programs competed with the rest of the industry. Attempts by the federal government to curb costs by restricting payments for routine procedures translated into fewer patients and shorter stays, thus leaving more beds empty. Nursing homes, too, suffered as restrictions on public reimbursement for chronic care made these facilities more dependent on patients' ability to pay privately for services. Finally, home health agencies performed many of the services that hospice programs offered and therefore resented the intrusion on their turf.

Limited referrals made it difficult for hospice programs to maintain an adequate census, and providers employed several strategies to increase referrals, such as marketing hospice services. For example, Cody and Naierman (1990) described their efforts to develop a liaison system with staff at several hospitals. They were unsuccessful in their efforts to be included at hospital discharge planning meetings, but educating staff about which patients were appropriate for hospice care served to increase referrals by 17 percent.

Developing day care programs for the terminally ill and offering consulting services were other ways to increase referrals. Some states allocated funds for the development and support of day care programs, and in 1989 Medicare established reimbursement for hospice programs that provided day care. Some hospice programs suggested their expertise could be helpful to nursing home staff and marketed the hospice team as a consulting service that would train nursing home staff in terminal care methods. Hospice Care, Inc., of Pinellas Park, Florida, was among those who developed such services. This hospice program became the consultant for 60 out of 78 nursing homes in the area. Its target population was patients living in a nursing home who became terminally ill and those terminally ill patients living at home who needed nursing home care.

Finally, hospice services in America had traditionally been limited to cancer patients, but as providers struggled to increase referrals, some suggested that the holistic and humanistic qualities of hospice care could benefit patients and families coping with such life-threatening illnesses as ALS (Lou Gehrig's disease) and Alzheimer's. These advocates pointed to Saint Christopher's Hospice in England, where all patients, regardless of diagnosis, had access to hospice care.

**The Failure to Effect the Ideal Components of Care** The ideal components of care determined early on by hospice advocates included pain management, spiritual support, and bereavement support. As the movement reached maturity it became clear that these goals had not been achieved. Although hospice advocates in the 1980s often claimed to be providing the "good death" that was key to hospice philosophy, such claims were largely supported by the clientele being served rather than any real difference in treatment between hospice care and conventional care.

Admission procedures to hospice programs favored elderly, middle-class, terminally ill patients with supportive families (Mor 1985). By delivering services to predominantly elderly clients who were more complacent about death and by insisting on a personal care provider, a number of programs were able to provide the "good death" that was central to hospice philosophy.

Efforts to fight against cure-at-all-costs methods of medical care were not evident. Patients receiving hospice care services might still receive aggressive treatments in the hope that they would have some impact, and hospice staff were reluctant to oppose personal physicians; at best they circumvented them. Being used to expedite discharge or compensate for poor hospital staffing were common complaints from hospice providers who wanted to do more.

Moreover, although hospice programs were numerous, these providers served only a minority of terminally ill patients (Rhymes 1990). Research found that terminally ill cancer patients had more unmet needs than did cancer patients who were newly diagnosed (Houts, Yasko, Harvey, Kahn, et al. 1988). The problems encountered by these terminally ill cancer patients were lack of in-home assistance, physical or emotional support, and financial assistance—services hospice programs were supposed to provide.

Various researchers (Kane 1986; Kastenbaum 1991; McCusker 1984; Zimmer, Groth and McCusker 1984) found that hospice care providers were no more successful at reducing pain than were traditional health care programs. Pain control and symptom management that emphasized physical treatment were overvalued by the movement's leaders, and other aspects of pain control, such as talking to patients and helping them cope with their anxiety, were downplayed in America (Klagsbrun 1982; Torrens 1985).

Early providers of hospice care had been particularly interested in reforming pain management for the terminal cancer patient, but there was little evidence that hospice programs improved the situation. Some physicians, despite the growing interest in research on pain control, were still hesitant to prescribe narcotics around the clock because they believed that administering drugs in this way resulted in tolerance for drugs or addiction (Rhymes 1990; Ufema 1989). Research regarding pain management was still in its early stages, and researchers questioned the effectiveness and the high cost of using barbiturates in the manner prescribed by Saunders (Foley 1989). Moreover, hospice teams were not always well trained in pain management and symptom control techniques, and therefore they could neither advocate nor provide proper treatment (Ufema 1989).

Spiritual support services, never backed by policymakers, were notably absent across the board. Amenta (1988) asserted that reports from program providers and hospice surveyors nationwide indicated that "spiritual care is one of the weakest hospice program elements" (47).

Research indicated that 40 percent of programs were noncompliant or only partially compliant in providing spiritual services (McCann 1985). Caregivers avoided providing pastoral care, and spirituality was ill defined in hospice programs (Millison and Dudley 1990). Nurses were not always able to distinguish spiritual distress from emotional distress. Pastoral care also suffered because providers tended to be tuned into their own religious philosophy (a sectarian approach) or took a watered-down counseling approach (Mount 1985). Moreover, only 1 percent of the hospice literature was about the spiritual aspects of care (Dush 1988).

There are a number of suppositions as to why little attention was paid to these services. One possible explanation is that Americans became uninterested in spirituality and therefore did not seek these services, even on their deathbed. Others suggest that the spiritual component of hospice care in England was due largely to Saunders's spirituality (Holden 1978); her program could be replicated, but her spirituality could not (Klagsbrun 1982).

Finally, to understand the limited attention given to spiritual support, we must look at pastoral caregivers as a collective force. Although key players in the development of early programs, religious leaders did not emphasize spiritual services. As newer programs emerged nurses provided pastoral services, and they did not seek out the assistance of local clergy (McCann 1985). Ministers did not protest when nurses usurped their position on hospice teams. In effect, clergy supported hospice care, but they did not seek legitimization for themselves.

Bereavement support, according to hospice philosophy, was an equally important aspect of patient care, but the average program spent only $83 dollars per client on bereavement services. Freestanding programs spent only $23. This amount represented only 1 percent of the programs' total service costs (Kidder 1987). Given such poor funding, the services offered were limited. Psychologists were rarely members of hospice teams (Lentz and Ramsey 1988). Although counseling was the most commonly offered service aside from nursing, it was volunteers who provided such support (Dush 1988).

For most providers bereavement services meant phone contacts and nursing visits (Kidder 1987; Kriebel 1989; Latanzi-Licht 1989). Anecdotal accounts indicated that there was little documentation or research on the impact of bereavement services and that some services appeared to be the poor stepchild of hospice programs (Latanzi-Licht 1989). The majority of programs had no full-time bereavement coordinator; any member of the team might be responsible for providing bereavement services. Volunteers, who were most often the ones to do so, felt ill prepared to help families (Byrd and Taylor 1989). Not surprisingly, research on bereavement services found that hospice care did not reduce survivors' morbidity or mortality (Parkes 1979), nor did it seem to significantly influence survivors' grief reactions (Beckwith, Beckwith, Gray, et al. 1990; Kane, Wales, Bernstein, Leibowitz, and Kaplan 1984).

Easing professional caregivers' stress was another ideal component of hospice care. Newer programs saw the weekly staff meetings initially advocated by movement participants an inefficient use of time, given the constraints of reimbursement. Tehan (1985) questioned the validity of spending staff time in this way; if staff members were not tied up in meetings they could be taking care of patients and billing insurers.

Although an estimated 71 percent of programs had weekly meetings, the content or quality of such meetings was not examined (Mor, Greer, and Kastenbaum 1988).

## Evaluating Hospice Care

First and foremost hospice researchers assert that there is a lack of research on hospice care (Dush 1988; Lamers 1988; Mount 1985; Paradis 1988). Seale (1989), assessing the trends in hospice care, noted that the National Hospice Study conducted from 1980 to 1982 was the only large-scale research into hospice care's benefits. Content analysis of the literature conducted in 1985 found that 24 percent of the articles were about the hospice concept, cost, and management. Most of the remaining articles were about issues related to hospice care, such as discussion of death and dying (12 percent), psychosocial issues (10 percent), and stress and burnout (10 percent) (Dush 1988).

The bulk of the literature was descriptive; evaluations of different hospice program types or of their influence on dying patients and their families were inadequate. Moreover, empirical research had a bias; researchers studied hospice programs that fit their definition of hospice—the medically oriented hospice program—and ignored community volunteer programs.

The National Hospice Study, sponsored by the Health Care Financing Administration and conducted by a group at Brown University in Rhode Island (Greer, et al. 1986) assessed 25 demonstration hospice programs, 14 nondemonstration hospice programs, and 14 conventional care programs. This study found, as did another smaller study (Kane, et al. 1984), that little difference existed between hospice care and traditional methods of care.

Specifically, the study found that hospice care did little to reduce pain or improve quality of life. Costs for hospice services varied according to program type. All programs were cheaper than traditional health care services if the time span for patient care was not extensive. Patients who received hospice services for a long time, however, incurred higher costs than did their nonhospice counterparts.

In some instances hospice care, according to this same study, reduced family stress and health care costs. Families who received inpatient hospice services experienced less stress during a patient's final illness than did nonhospice patients. Furthermore, the National Hospice Study found that survivors were less likely than the national norm to experience secondary morbidity (illness resulting from grief); this study also found, however, that families who did not have access to inpatient care experienced more distress after death.

Anecdotal observations and small studies of hospice services were mixed as to whether hospice programs benefitted from their affiliation with hospitals or were adversely affected. Some anecdotal accounts suggested that being a legitimate, integral part of the traditional health care system would help hospice programs continue to grow and develop (Munley 1983; Paradis and Cummings 1986; Tehan 1985). Other studies of selected aspects of hospice care found programs falling short of ideals (Corless 1985; Hoyer 1990; Greer and Mor 1985; Kulys and Davis 1986; Mount 1985).

Limitations regarding pain management, bereavement counseling, and spiritual support have been discussed already, but there were many other weaknesses identified by researchers. Among these problems were staff stress as the result of working with dying patients, insurers' lack of interest in funding this form of care, and difficulty in providing a full complement of services. Diagnostic activities were more common in scatter-bed models (Hannon and O'Donnell 1984), and, although hospice patients were more likely than nonhospice patients to receive psychosocial services, access varied widely among the types of hospice (Mor 1987).

Mount (1985) asserted that hospices had not performed up to optimal levels and that the responsibility for this lay with the groups providing hospice care. "North American studies of terminal care suggest both an intrinsic deficiency and a general lack of perception of that deficiency by the caregivers involved. Both aspects of the problem are significant since change will only be evoked and improvements in care promoted when those responsible for health care are convinced that there is a serious need that demands attention" (22). He added that the enthusiasm regarding the popular appeal of hospice care and motivation to become a part of this service overshadowed limitations in training and subsequent limitations on the way that services were provided.

As has been noted, hospice care seemed to favor an educated, middle-class clientele. Consequently, there were many terminally ill people who did not receive hospice services. The following sections describe two groups, minority and rural patients, who were identified as having inadequate access to hospice services.

**Minorities and Hospice Care**   Minority patients were rarely the recipients of hospice services. The National Hospice Study found that 91.6 percent of patients receiving services were white and non-Hispanic (Mor and Hiris 1983). Smaller studies reflected a similar trend (Buckingham and Lupu 1982; Creek 1982). Some pointed to government funding (Wald 1989) or inadequate medical staff training (Lescohier 1990) as the reasons that minorities—as well as the poor—did not receive hospice care. But research indicated that the organization and philosophy of the hospice programs contributed to discrimination against minorities. Hospice programs were organized and run by whites, and hospice conferences were predominantly attended by white females (Neubauer and Hamilton 1990). Moreover, minorities may have been excluded to prevent any controversy from slowing the movement: "Has hospice used the expedient of excluding minority persons to avoid additional controversy and gain power and structural approval" (Meyers 1990, 19)?

Robert Butler (personal communication) suggested that hospice care was essentially a middle-class phenomenon that emerged as an educated public became interested in the psychology of death and dying. Hospice services might not be desirable to minorities. Research found that African-Americans, for example, "were more likely to want to live as long as possible under almost any circumstances and more likely to think that death should be avoided at all costs" (Neubauer and Hamilton 1990, 44).

**Rural Hospice Programs**   Rural hospice programs were slower in getting started because of problems in adapting the concept to rural areas (Coordinating Council for Independent Living 1986). These programs were smaller, with few staff and patients, but they had to service large geographic areas. Providers in rural areas claimed that Medicare regulations discriminated against them (Wakefield, Curry, and Kieffer 1987). Medicare not only provided inadequate reimbursement for services, it also expected staff to provide all direct services.

Rural programs were often too small to support a separate professional team. Moreover, professionals were a scarce resource in rural areas. Census studies found that urban counties were more likely to have Medicare-approved hospice programs than nonurban counties (Hoyer 1990). Missouri and West Virginia, two predominantly rural states, did not apply for reimbursement because they believed Medicare structures undermined the quality of care and placed providers in too much financial jeopardy (Coordinating Council for Independent Living 1986; Shanis 1985).

Rural areas that affiliated with urban-suburban centers were in a better position to utilize Medicare certification, but this created other access problems. Research on hospice programs serving rural Pennsylvanians (Siebold and Bucher 1990) found that families did not have equal access to services. The providers studied by these researchers tended to be tied to large medical structures that have historically offered inadequate services to rural people. Agencies were nurse dominated, located in suburban centers, and emphasized physical care. Other staff were either shared with larger systems, such as home health agencies, or they were consultants.

According to this Pennsylvania study, the more geographically isolated the patient, the greater the difficulty in providing services. Service provision was designed based on reimbursement; therefore, time and cost prevented providers from offering in-home support in hard-to-reach areas. The farther away the patient was geographically from the agency, the more likely it was that a nurse would provide all direct services, such as emotional support, physical therapy, and social services. Moreover, nursing interventions were often carried out by phone, and some patients living in isolated areas were refused admission to hospice programs.

Rural communities traditionally depended on local volunteers to compensate for the lack of available professional staff, and Jenkins and Cook (1981) asserted that because hospice programs used volunteers they were a natural fit with rural tradition. Siebold and Bucher (1990), however, found that volunteers were not a stable resource for rural patients; providers reported that they had difficulty finding volunteers willing to travel to hard-to-reach places, and some providers felt that volunteers did not have the professional skills to provide adequate hospice services.

Other limitations in the Pennsylvania programs surveyed were the availability of narcotics, bereavement services, and access to inpatient respite care. Some rural physicians were reluctant to prescribe around-the-clock barbiturates, and rural pharmacies did not always provide 24-hour service. Access to inpatient hospital beds was limited; 44 percent of hospice programs reported using nursing home beds some of the time, 27 percent reported using nursing homes exclusively, and 18 percent had no inpatient respite services. Furthermore, the majority of programs provided little in the way of bereavement services; only 3 out of 20 (18 percent) conducted some form of counseling for survivors.

Several references have been made to the lack of political support within the movement for spiritual services, yet this rural survey found that clergy were always available to volunteer their services to hospice patients. The ministry was carrying out its traditional function, meeting the needs of the terminally ill and their families regardless of the organizational structure under which they served.

**Current Trends**  It would be unfair to those professionals and volunteers who continue asserting the original intent of the hospice movement to suggest that collective activities to alter conditions for the dying in this country have ceased. They have not. They are less evident, however, and there are signs that the American hospice movement is no longer as vigorous as it was during the mid-1970s and early 1980s. To its credit, the movement established programs that provide greater assistance to families than existed in the past, and most families appreciate the in-home supports that they receive.

The following paragraphs give examples of the dominant political trends of the movement—integration with medical environments and reduction of services to survivors. Seale (1989) asserted that although hospice philosophy had influenced traditional medical care slightly, the traditional health care system was more likely to co-opt and deflect hospice services. In Maine, until 1991, programs were staffed by volunteers, and these providers did not participate in the hospice movement's political process. Local ministers, nurses, and other concerned individuals who wanted to alleviate the emotional, spiritual, and physical distress that families and patients experienced during a terminal illness created a service structure based on hospice principles. By 1991, however, providers began to formalize these services and seek Medicare funding. Given the restrictions of Medicare and the medicalizing trends that are associated with seeking such reimbursement, it is likely that physical care needs and the traditional medical model may soon alter the spirit of these programs. To their credit, these providers are aware of such dangers and are attempting to preserve the programs' humanistic qualities.

Perhaps even more poignant is the closing of Saint Luke's Hospice in New York City. As the reader will remember, Saint Luke's was the second hospice program to develop in this country and the first scatter-bed model. This program integrated hospice programs with the acute health care system and advocated the importance of pain management and symptom control. Concurrently, it also was a spirited opponent of the personal care provider ruling, and minorities made up the majority of its patient population (Pawling-Kaplan and O'Connor 1989). Medicare funding was inadequate to support inpatient services, and the program depended on private donations and hospital support to maintain its professional team.

Public support from hospice leaders such as Tom West, medical director at Saint Christopher's in England, who asserted the importance of continuing Saint Luke's palliative care program, was not enough to preserve this hospice program. In 1991 funding restrictions forced Saint Luke's palliative care program to close.

## Conclusion

Hospice care providers had assumed that theirs was a popular cause that was sure to succeed. The movement's leaders emphasized funding needs and tolerated variations to increase the number of programs. Research regarding who was served by hospice care and what was reimbursed by policymakers indicated that leaders' assumptions were inaccurate. The public did not crave hospice services; in fact, people were unaware of what a hospice program did. Moreover, policymakers had used hospice programs for other purposes, particularly reducing costs, and most programs failed to provide a service that was substantially different from other health care services.

As Medicare regulations came into being, what had been a peaceful coexistence among leaders and participants became a battleground of different interest groups who were unwilling to compromise. A fragmentation process occurred whereby some programs conformed to the dominant political forces of the time, others went their own way, and a few held onto their original ideals. Ultimately, the cost of services was much greater than participants had anticipated, and the financial support from the government was anything but generous.

*Chapter 8*

# The Movement's Accomplishments

The consequences of a social movement are greater than its obvious accomplishments or failings. Leaders' abilities to institute new programs or policies are the best known outcomes of social movements, yet the social forces at work within them also influence cultural values and beliefs.

The creation of a nationwide network of hospice programs, funded by Medicare, Medicaid, and other health insurers, was the movement's best-known achievement. But there were several other ways that attitudes toward, and treatment of, the dying were influenced. Hospice philosophy affected staff attitudes regarding patients' needs and the provision of terminal care. Modern hospice programs were timely; they provided a method of care appropriate for AIDS patients and children who suffered from cancer. Moreover, as an international movement, the hospice concept has spread to many different cultures.

## Influences on Terminal Care

Despite the problems hospice providers faced as they tried to create programs, the hospice movement did influence the health care system. Services provided by individual programs might not be completely in keeping with the movement's original goals, but they represented an alternative form of terminal care. Dying patients were more likely to receive nonaggressive, supportive health care services, and they could die in the presence of family and friends.

164

Whether patients received hospice services or not, there was greater acceptance that death at home was an option. Communication about death was no longer tabu; discussing prognosis with patients was acknowledged as an important pursuit by health care providers. Moreover, nurses, the clergy, and social workers, as part of the health care team, were allowed to encourage patients and families to discuss their feelings and treatment options.

Providing a network of hospice services reduced waiting lists at older terminal care facilities. For example, Calvary Hospital, one of the few hospitals in the country that specializes in care of terminally ill cancer patients, found that the rise in hospice programs reduced their referrals. Before 1975 requests for beds at Calvary were far greater than the hospital's capacity; patients often died in another hospital awaiting transfer. The increase in hospice services resulted in fewer referrals (Cimino 1983, 225).

The philosophy of hospice care was not restricted to the network of programs so named. As hospice programs experienced difficulty surviving because of financial and regulatory constraints, other programs were created that espoused hospice philosophy but used a different name. "Although the hospice movement has grown, many areas of the country have not adopted the formal governmental hospice definition" (Yancy and Grieger 1990, 24). In Indiana a hospital-based extended care facility developed the Mary Margaret Center, which consisted of suites for families and patients. The suites allowed them to stay in a homelike setting, but with nursing staff available on a 24-hour basis.

A subtler influence of hospice philosophy is evidenced by the development of cancer care programs that are affiliated with hospital services but do not consider themselves hospices. For example, the Cancer Support Service in Maine provides nursing care and psychosocial support for patients with terminal cancer, but there are restrictions on neither life expectancy nor the forms of treatment the patient can receive. Rather, these providers determine with patients and families what options are available and support them in whatever decision they make.

Pain management techniques also transcended programs and became part of medical treatment. "Certainly hospice has sparked research into the badly neglected area of pain control" (Sherman and Finn 1987, 379). For example, a national conference on health and the control of pain held in 1979 yielded numerous papers on pain studies and principles of terminal care (Abdellah, Harper, Lunceford 1982). At another conference, Peter

Bourne, White House advisor on health, asserted the need for research on pain management in 1978.

> We have convened the Interagency Committee on New Therapies for Pain and Discomfort to establish a national policy for the treatment of those in pain and the terminally ill. The membership of the Committee includes representatives from the National Institute on Aging, the Food and Drug Administration, Health Resources Administration, National Institute for Mental Health, and the Drug Enforcement Administration, as well as representatives from the Committee on the Treatment of Intractable Pain, the National Academy of Sciences, Institute of Medicine and members of Congress. This varied membership illustrates both the need for coordination and the great amount of interest that has already developed on this important issue. The focus of the Committee is broad and their inquiry will not be limited to the use of Heroin or Cannabis. Rather they will foster research on developing better methods for treatment of death, dying, and chronic pain, including all forms of therapy not just chemotherapy. They will look at mechanics of pain, see that research findings are shared widely and promote a coherent government policy toward the treatment of the terminally ill. (*Hospice Newsletter*, June 1978)

Although inpatient hospice services, particularly Saint Christopher's, had the greatest success in managing chronic pain, better pain management was becoming part of all health care services (Gotay 1983). In England, "Retrospective study of the relatives' assessment of pain control indicates that patients suffered less distress and less pain in 1977–79 compared with 1967–69 and suggests that hospital staffs have learned new skills." (Ford 1984, 211). Recent American studies of all forms of hospice programs find that these programs often do not provide better pain control than does traditional health services; a partial explanation for this is that pain management was picked up by mainstream medicine (Seale 1989).[4]

## Hospice Care for Children

By the late 1970s interest developed in England and America in the special problems of terminally ill children and their families. Health care workers emerged to champion this cause, and they created model hospice programs for children. Like their predecessors, who had developed adult hospice programs, those asserting the need for pediatric hospice care struggled to acquire resources such as staff, education, and funds. Advocating children's hospices had an advantage, however, in having witnessed the problems associated with creating adult programs.

At the Second Annual Conference on Hospice Care in 1977 in Riverside, New Jersey, providers noted that a few programs had begun providing services for children. These first services were not separate programs but were part of existing adult programs. The Hospice of Marin, for example, provided home care services for children as well as adults. The first hospice programs specializing in the care of children with terminal illnesses did not get started until the early 1980s. Saint Mary's Hospice in Bayside, Queens, and Melinda House in Washington, D.C., were among the first, and they offered inpatient and home care services.

During the late 1970s studies were conducted to assess the needs of terminally ill children and the practicalities of creating hospice programs for them. Ida Martinson (Ewens and Herrington 1983), a nurse educator, researched the benefits of home care hospice services for children and families in Minnesota; at Saint Mary's Hospital in New York researchers conducted a feasibility study (Wilson 1982). Researchers interviewed hospice and pediatric experts, assessed demographic data, studied funding sources, and evaluated potential referral patterns.

Generally speaking, researchers found that terminally ill children were unlike adults; the range of illnesses afflicting children differed, as did the physical and emotional impact these illnesses had on them. Leukemia, brain tumors, muscular dystrophy, and cystic fibrosis (and, during the 1980s, AIDS) were the most common terminal diseases of childhood. Pain control for children was unstudied, and lifespan was more difficult to predict. Additionally, the degree of emotional trauma for family and caregivers was greater than in the case of an adult's death.

Experts reported that fear of death was not natural to children but was instilled in them by parents. Therefore, hospice services could provide an environment of open communication where death was not a hidden, secretive, and fearful experience. They also asserted the need for greater family supports by hospice providers.

The death of a baby is shattering. The death of a child with whom the parents have become acquainted and for whom long-range plans have been made can be even more traumatic. In this situation, the relationship between the parents is often at stake. Studies have shown that a large number of parents separate following the death of their child (70 percent in one study, 90 percent in another), whereas with support that percentage can be significantly reduced (to 7 percent in one study). (Wilson 1982, 207–8)

Hospice services would benefit children and parents because dying children could remain in their own homes, where they felt safe and where family members felt greater control. Because family control and open communication were so important, developers of children's hospice programs asserted that they had to take care to prevent these programs from becoming subsumed by mainstream medicine, as had been the case with many adult hospice programs. Finally, the number of children requiring services would not be great; during the first year providers would need to study patient census patterns and plan accordingly.

Careful assessment of the problems of terminally ill children and their families resulted in the establishment of hospice programs that were more in tune with consumers' needs. All chronically ill children were eligible. Because most parents wanted to keep their child at home but required daytime assistance, day programs were popular components of children's hospice services. Neonatal intensive care units were another service that utilized the hospice concept. These units emphasized prolonging the infant's life, regardless of the degree of impairment or long-term prognosis. Because medical technology sustains life but often cannot undo the extraordinary physical damage these infants are born with, acute care providers acknowledged a need for assistance to help parents and staff decide when to turn the machines off. Hospice workers in such units were able to provide families and staff with the emotional support needed to make these difficult decisions and to grieve their loss (Spiegel 1982).

Despite the interest in hospices for children, few programs were created. By 1983 there were fewer than 20 programs, and program form was not uniform; different program types were created, such as a home care program in Louisville, Kentucky, a hospital-based program in Milwaukee, and a hospital-affiliated community service in Los Angeles.

Researchers asserted that one reason there were fewer children's programs was that physicians and families were reluctant to acknowledge a child's terminal status (Buckingham and Loveday 1983). Another factor that impeded the development of children's hospices was the lack of established funding for such programs. Traditional insurance coverage was not adequate for the amount of services recommended for children, and it was often used up during the course of aggressive treatment. Hospice programs providing children's services found that parents had also depleted their financial reserves, were unable to pay for hospice services, and could not apply for Medicaid without jeopardizing the whole family's economic security. No federal policy emerged to address these problems, and hospices were therefore dependent on fund-raising and special grants to offset the cost of providing services.

A significant contributor to the effort to establish hospice services for children was Ann Armstrong Dailey. While studying medicine at Georgetown University, Dailey was approached by a family who wanted to keep their terminally ill child at home. The lack of services, however, made this impossible. Observing this family's struggle sensitized Dailey to this issue and led her to leave medical training to become an advocate of children's hospice care in the United States.

As a consequence of Dailey's efforts, in 1980 the Hospice of Northern Virginia began accepting children in its home care service. In 1983 Dailey founded and became the executive director of a nonprofit organization, Children's Hospice International (CHI) in Alexandria, Virginia. CHI's purpose was to study, educate, and establish an agenda regarding issues pertinent to terminal illness in children. "To raise money and support [for CHI], she [Dailey] criss-crossed the country, giving lectures and holding symposiums for hospice staff members, health-care professionals and the public. By 1986, CHI had provided education training and technical assistance to more than 100 hospice home care programs for children" (Phillips 1991, 38–39).

Dailey went on to create an independent hospice facility in 1989 for terminally ill children called Melinda House in the Washington, D.C., area, obtaining funds with the help of Milton Glatt, a child psychiatrist. Although the primary goal of Melinda House is to provide inpatient and home care services to dying children, "the second dimension of Melinda House is designed to promote the development and further acceptance of pediatric hospice care on international and national levels. The major aspects of this dimension will strengthen direct pediatric hospice care by promoting research, technical assistance, and advocacy of care for termi-nally ill children and their families. A library and resource center will be established at Melinda House that will be used for research and education" (Dailey and DiTullio 1988, 15).

**British Programs** The British experience of creating hospice programs for children was similar to America's. Children dying of advanced-stage diseases captured the attention of people working in hospice programs or pediatric care units, and these individuals became spokespersons for the needs of dying children. For example, a staff member at Saint Christopher's Hospice and a pediatrician who had worked with children dying of cystic fibrosis wrote of their experiences caring for terminally ill children, thus drawing attention to their plight and establishing that they had special needs (Chapman and Goodall 1979).

Another early advocate was Sister Frances Dominica, who trained as a pediatric nurse. She found that "however kind and skilled the staff were, one thing was clear; this was not the right setting for a child who was dying slowly. A hospital is too busy, too noisy, and where a choice must be made staff are necessarily more concerned with promoting recovery than tending the dying. The child's own home is surely the ideal setting" (Farrow 1981, 1433).

Sister Frances set out in the early 1980s to build a special facility, Helen House, in Oxford, England. Helen House was named after a little girl who had suffered a brain tumor at the age of two and whose parents had been determined to care for her at home, but needed respite services. The architectural design of Helen House reflected the special needs of dying children.

> At Helen House there will be eight rooms, each with a bed and a window seat that converts into a divan for a parent to sleep beside the child. Several of the rooms can be opened out to create two-bed "wards." There are also two double-bedrooms with attendant facilities for parents to stay. There will be a hydrotherapy pool, and hobby and play/study rooms. There is a garden and outdoor play area. (Farrow 1981, 1434)

Financing for the facility did not come from the British National Health Service. Local sources and public donations provided the funds to create and sustain Helen House, and families contributed to the cost of care if they chose to. Helen House became a model program imitated by other providers seeking to create children's hospice programs.

**Children and AIDS** During the early 1980s the AIDS epidemic became a concern for hospice advocates. Children with AIDS, like adult AIDS patients, faced discriminatory practices. Hospital administrators were reluctant to provide services for AIDS patients, often out of fear that other clients would stay away from a hospital admitting persons with AIDS (Dailey 1988).

Families of these children coped with a special set of circumstances. The duration of the disease was unpredictable; infants might survive for a few months or for years. A family member was often responsible for the

child's having contracted the disease. Children were usually infected peri-
natally; they were born with the HIV virus because their parent was
infected. Other children contracted the disease because of sexual abuse.
Finally, a minority of children contracted the disease from blood transfusions. Families were often secretive about their children's illnesses
because they feared the discrimination and isolation that they and their
child would have to endure, but secrecy meant that they had to bear the
emotional and physical burden of the illness alone.

Based on these issues, hospice advocates asserted that admission criteria for children with AIDS should be amended. Criteria such as a six-
month prognosis or cessation of aggressive treatments were impractical
for these children and their families. Children with AIDS required early
admission to receive adequate support, and deserved any potential benefits
from experimental treatments, such as AZT. Finally, because many of the
children who suffered from AIDS had parents who were themselves sick
or dead, foster homes or special housing was particularly important. The
lack of supportive families and/or inpatient hospice facilities meant children with AIDS spending much of their life in acute care hospitals.

The thrust of pediatric hospice care advocates was to take a proactive
position in designing services for children with AIDS, and their efforts
had some success. For example, in 1989 Melinda House began providing
assistance to children with AIDS, and Children's Hospice International
acted as a clearinghouse for information regarding children and AIDS.
The Abandoned Infants Assistance Act, passed in October 1988, was the
first federal policy that supported the establishment of children's inpatient
hospice facilities.

## Response to the AIDS Epidemic

The AIDS epidemic mobilized some hospice advocates to reassert the
movement's ideals. At the 1985 National Hospice Organization's Annual
Conference in Washington, D.C., NHO representatives stated that hospice
providers should make services available to AIDS patients. But they never
mandated the expansion of hospice services. Hospice providers' response
to the disease was mixed. Some provided services for these patients as a
matter of course, while others, who were struggling to survive, welcomed
this new patient population. Many providers, however, resisted including
AIDS patients on their caseload.

Within the hospice movement leaders and providers of services were quick to assert the need to assist persons with AIDS. Elisabeth Kübler-Ross attempted to create services for AIDS patients, and she encouraged open communication about the disease. The symptoms of AIDS, however, were different from those of other terminal diseases and required greater investigation. Cicely Saunders asserted that PWAs should be treated in separate facilities by teams that specialized in managing the physical and psychosocial issues related to AIDS. Certain hospice providers, such as the Visiting Nurse Association of San Francisco and Saint Vincent's Hospital in New York, both of which cared for terminally ill cancer patients, also became specialists in managing care of AIDS patients. They trained others regarding the special needs of this group.

The first program developers implemented their ideas amidst communities' fears of having AIDS facilities in their neighborhoods. For example, a group of religious women opened an AIDS hospice in Washington, D.C., in 1985, but only after overcoming the local community's fear of persons with AIDS. Kübler-Ross also started an AIDS facility, but she too struggled against community resistance. One group in New York was thwarted in its attempts to use a building to house AIDS patients because a landmark commission asserted that the building had been the the residence of composer Anton Dvorak and therefore should be preserved as a historical site, not converted into an AIDS hospice.

Although AIDS patients represented the potential for increased referrals, most hospice programs were as inflexible as traditional health care systems in their ability to alter rules to overcome policies that restricted AIDS patients' eligibility for services. A 1990 survey of programs in New York found that these providers had yet to serve AIDS patients (Wilkinson, MacDonald, and Pelz 1990). Persons with AIDS often did not have a personal care person, were not covered by Medicare or Medicaid, and were younger and unwilling to give up aggressive treatments (Wallace 1990). Furthermore, the complexity of symptoms that accompanied the immune deficiency disease and the stigma of the disease (Kidder 1987) made AIDS patients unpopular with many providers. Many home health hospice programs refused to accept AIDS patients.

Activists who observed that traditional health care providers were slow to respond to the needs of PWAs established their own services. In particular, the gay community did not wait for outside support; instead they developed support groups, legal advocates, and in-home supports for AIDS sufferers. The Gay Men's Task Force in New York was one group that oversaw and participated in the creation of numerous services for AIDS patients.

AIDS victims were angry, not only because their life was ending but because society was unconcerned with helping to treat or find a cure for the disease. Although secrecy about their disease was a common phenomenon among AIDS victims, there also were members of the gay community who were willing to speak out to contest the discriminatory practices experienced by AIDS victims. Larry Kramer (1989), for example, wrote a series of articles about the experiences of gay men dying from AIDS and about the political processes responsible for the inadequate funding of research and treatment.

PWAs also participated in designing new hospice programs, thus making these services more congruent with patients' perceptions of need. Separate conferences about hospice care for AIDS patients were held. "The Hospice Response to AIDS," held in San Francisco in April 1988, covered topics such as understanding the AIDS epidemic, outreach to patients suffering from AIDS, and differences in providing care for AIDS patients. As had been the case with the early meetings of participants in the hospice movement, providers who had some experience in service provision presented their experience and advice to groups hoping to develop programs for AIDS patients.

**AIDS and Hospice Philosophy** The emergence of the AIDS epidemic, and humanitarians' response to it, caused a resurgence of many of the hospice movement's original ideals regarding patient control over their experience and patient and family being treated as a unit of care. Because PWAs experienced many assaults from society, control of their experience became an important concern (Touhey 1989). Moreover, families of PWAs required greater assistance than did those coping with the death of an elderly relative.

The right to information about prognosis, control over treatment cessation, and determination of place of death had been part of the original agenda of the hospice movement. Cancer patients never assembled to assert the importance of these concepts, and caregivers who believed they knew what was best made decisions for patients. PWAs were less willing to give control of their care over to health care workers. Unlike most cancer patients, who are elderly and often accustomed to leaving decisions about treatment to physicians, many AIDS patients in the 1980s were young, affluent, gay men who did not trust the medical establishment, and they demanded greater control over the services they received.

Providers who worked with AIDS patients and their families asserted that the various emotional themes that emerged were both similar to and different from those associated with other terminal illnesses. The experience of loss and the fear of death were common themes for all people facing terminal illness. AIDS patients and their families, however, also coped with homophobia, fear of contagion and stigma, and secrecy about the illness (Giacquinta 1989). Moreover, PWAs came from distinct social groups that faced different problems. Gay men coping with the spread of this disease experienced problems different from IV drug users or hemophiliacs. One experience they all shared, however, was that of the stigma attached to their disease.

Mourners, too, were unable to talk about their experience because of public prejudice. Friends might not empathize with their loss but rather judge them for having caused the disease or associated with an AIDS sufferer. Grief counseling was complicated.

Symptom control for AIDS patients quickly became specialized. Infection control was particularly important to protect PWAs from further exposure to opportunistic infections. AIDS added a new dimension to symptom management, helping patients cope with AIDS Related Complex (ARC), which results when the virus infects the central nervous system. The symptoms of AIDS dementia, for example, are evidenced by problems in cognition, reduced motor control, agitation, depression, psychosis, paralysis, seizures, and total personality change. Patients suffering from AIDS dementia required greater assistance, including homemaking and personal care services and counseling for themselves and their significant others. Ongoing peer support for staff and volunteers who worked with these patients was also needed (Carwein and Longley 1989).

The importance of volunteers in the patient care process had diminished in most hospice programs for cancer patients, but because many traditional health care systems shunned PWAs and because families and friends were often unavailable, volunteers again became an important source of support. At a hospice service in Amarillo, Texas, a training program was designed specifically for members of the gay and lesbian community who wanted to volunteer their services. Knight (1990) outlined the factors specific to training such volunteers.

Issues such as the volunteer's sense of identification with the PWA, losses the volunteer may have experienced within his own circle of friends, internalized homophobia, and specific psycho-social issues faced by the PWA need to be incorporated into the program's traditional training format. The unique aspects of grief experienced by members of the gay community also need to be examined. (32)

Initially, public funding for medical services to AIDS patients was limited, and services depended on fund-raising. In this environment, programs for infected members of the gay community fared better than did inner-city services for IV drug users. Discriminatory practices by insurers and employers toward AIDS sufferers were common. Medicaid reimbursed for services, but applying for Medicaid was a complicated process; moreover, patients had to be destitute to qualify. Medicare benefits also were of little assistance because most PWAs died before they became eligible for coverage. As the number of people infected with the virus continued to increase, advocacy groups were created to fight discriminatory practices and to appeal to legislators for special funds for AIDS services.

One subject that was missing from hospice providers' discussions about AIDS patients was the growing interest in assisted death, which became popular in the gay community during the mid-1980s. PWAs who had witnessed the effects of the disease on others and who realized that death was the inevitable outcome of the disease began seeking ways to commit suicide—active euthanasia—to avoid the discomfort and ignominy of the dying process. Hospice literature has had little to say about this topic, focusing instead on how to live until death and how to help patients and families cope with the emotional trauma resulting from the disease.

**Hospice Programs for AIDS Patients** As hospitals became over-crowded with AIDS patients who no longer needed acute inpatient treatment but whose families were unaware of their condition or were unable to care for them, alternatives were created. In San Francisco, where many PWAs were affluent men from the gay community, an early response resulted in the creation of good-quality hospice services for PWAs. The Shanti project, the San Francisco AIDS Foundation, and the Hospice of San Francisco were among these first programs. Other cities had greater difficulty orchestrating such an effective response (Edmondson 1990).

The Connecticut Hospice, Inc. (formerly Hospice, Inc.), began admitting AIDS patients in 1984. They were concerned about contagion, however, and initially restricted AIDS patients to private rooms. Staff took precautions such as donning masks and gloves before entering patients' rooms. Several years later, when the disease was better understood, AIDS patients were permitted to leave their rooms and join other patients in activities programs. Connecticut Hospice staff discovered that although AIDS patients often stabilized and could be discharged, they had no place to go. In response Hospice Cottage, a residence on hospital grounds, was opened for such individuals.

PWAs were frequently evicted from their homes or shut out by family and friends. Independent hospice buildings thus became an important component of care for AIDS patients. Open communication about death was common at AIDS facilities; in fact, it was encouraged. When a patient died at Casey House, a 17-bed palliative and acute care facility in Toronto, the body remained at the facility for a time to give residents the opportunity to acknowledge the death, and staff encouraged residents to talk about their memories of the person (Trent 1988).

Although the number of elderly people who contracted AIDS—as well as the number of young people who survived long enough to be eligible for Medicare reimbursement—was small, a group in Boston opened the first Medicare-certified AIDS hospice. This was a row house in Boston's Mission Hill district that was remodeled to become a 16-bed hospice facility. One custom of this facility that was common to many such hospices was the Remembrance Book; a picture book of all the people who had stayed at the hospice before their death (Tischler 1990).

Hospice programs that expanded to include PWAs soon found that admission criteria for other hospice patients were not applicable to AIDS patients. Hospice Care of Rhode Island began a program for AIDS patients in 1985, but after several months realized that admission requirements excluded most AIDS patients. In particular, admissions policies regarding life expectancy and cessation of active treatment were not appropriate for PWAs, and so they exempted PWAs from criteria. They also found that if they wanted to provide AIDS patients with services they had to interact with AIDS coalitions created to counteract the suspicion and secrecy that made PWAs reluctant to avail themselves of resources (McDuff, Toms, Gordon, and Rehm 1990).

As the number of people infected with the disease increased, communities could no longer presume that they would escape the AIDS epidemic, and the need for hospice services increased. In Kansas City, for example, the SAVE Foundation was created to provide inpatient and support services for poor AIDS victims. Funding for the program came from private contributions and community support. In Louisiana, as in Rhode Island, groups providing hospice care found that they were only one of a network of services designed to help PWAs. The Louisiana Aids Community Network (LACN) was an advocacy group that coordinated services such as hospice care, housing support, educational groups, and volunteer support systems (Kutzen 1986).

Another category of AIDS patients, IV drug users, required different services. IV drug users who contracted AIDS usually were not affluent people who could mobilize support groups or demand better services; public policy changes were required to influence access to services for this population. In 1986, policymakers in New York began exploring the idea of designating certain hospitals as AIDS centers and providing them with funds for comprehensive services. By 1989, 14 hospitals had been selected as AIDS centers, with as many other facilities applying for such designation. These centers functioned primarily to integrate aggressive, palliative, and psychosocial services that met the needs of patients and families. Reimbursement for outpatient services, the main thrust of these programs, was seven-tiered; fees for services were based on degree of difficulty and the expertise required.

(A curious twist in the development of programs for AIDS sufferers came as a result of sentencing criminal offenders to community service in lieu of prison sentences; providing AIDS services was one way to fulfill this sentence. For example, a man sentenced for dealing drugs might opt to manage an AIDS residence. Hospice participants had mixed opinions about this new method of service provision. Galazka expressed concern that hospices were being used for alternative sentencing: "This can send the wrong message to the public; working with PWAs and cancer patients is equal to or worse than a prison sentence" [[1990, 18]. Caring for seriously ill patients, however, appears to have been meaningful for many [Klagsbrun 1982; Krant 1974].)

**Resistance to Hospice Programs for AIDS Patients** Community resistance to creating AIDS hospices is a common theme in the literature. In Canada, for example, an order of nuns known as Les Filles de la Charité was defeated in an effort to create an AIDS hospice. This order was established during the nineteenth century to alleviate social problems such as drug addiction and child abuse. When it inherited property in Martinville, Quebec, the order decided to convert the building into an AIDS hospice.

The project started when Sister Florence, who was given charge of the property, contacted a local social worker, Louise Lalonde, to discuss what kinds of services were needed in the Martinville community. Lalonde was in charge of finding foster homes to care for chronically or terminally ill patients; among her caseload were two AIDS patients whom she could not place. She told Sister Florence that an AIDS hospice was a desperately needed service.

Although Martinville's mayor and parish priest supported the idea, the town council and local citizens disagreed. They didn't believe the town needed such a facility, and they expressed many fears regarding the presence of PWAs in their community, such as fear of contagion and fear that property values would drop. Opposition to instituting a hospice spread and initial concerns were exaggerated; residents asserted that their community would be overrun with AIDS patients from all over, that the disease would infect their children, and that the town would no longer be fit to live in.

The fears that fueled citizen protest toward the project also led them to take action against those who supported it. They questioned the parish priest's commitment to the community, made threatening calls to Sister Florence, and criticized the few town residents who agreed to having an AIDS hospice. Public opinion was allowed to decide the question, even though legally the town council could not have stopped the sisters. The project was abandoned; instead the sisters opened a battered women's shelter.

## The International Hospice Movement

The needs of the terminally ill have inspired the development of special hospitals and programs throughout the world. The efforts of Mother Teresa in India, Father Chanley in Malaya, and the Madame Curie Foundation in London are examples of independent attempts to ameliorate conditions for dying people. An international hospice movement, however, inspired by Saint Christopher's Hospice and Cicely Saunders's modern hospice concept, was the greatest impetus for program creation around the world. In Australia, Canada, England, Ireland, Poland, South Africa, and West Germany hospices proliferated, and Saunders was asked to help create these new programs. By 1980, 16 countries were represented at an international conference on hospice care held in London.

**British Programs**  Hospices for the terminally ill have existed in England since the late nineteenth century and were more commonly known than hospices in America; but it was the opening of Saint Christopher's Hospice in 1967 that encouraged the spread of hospices throughout the United Kingdom. Hospices proliferated earlier in the United Kingdom than in other countries; by 1975 there more than 1,000 beds available and a demand that could have filled three times as many (Lamerton 1975). In contrast, American hospice advocates were just starting the first three programs and Canadians were creating their first program.

Since the 1970s, 111 inpatient facilities and 170 home care programs have opened in England, Wales, and Ireland. Aside from an earlier start, hospice developers in the United Kingdom also had greater access to financial support. The first hospices were developed independent of the National Health Service (NHS). They relied instead on endowments and public donations. The Marie Curie Foundation, the MacMillan Fund, and the National Society for Cancer were the major funding sources that established and sustained programs. In particular, the MacMillan Fund played a major role in the creation of the first hospices. This fund, established in 1911 by a Scotsman Douglas MacMillan, helped build the first modern independent facilities and provided training for hospice nurses (Gilmore 1989).

The preferred British model of hospice care was an independent facility that provided inpatient and home care services. A 1980 report by the National Society for Cancer, however, determined that high costs would make it difficult to continue creating inpatient facilities. Limited public donations and a reduced budget for the National Health Service limited the money available to support new construction. Subsequently, home care hospice teams and hospital support teams based on the American scatter-bed model at Saint Luke's Hospice became more common.

**British versus American Programs**  Hospice providers in the United Kingdom avoided or simply did not face some of the pitfalls encountered by their American counterparts. The former were especially concerned that hospice services not be dominated by the National Health Service, which might dilute the quality of services. American hospice programs struggled to obtain sufficient referrals, whereas British hospice programs could not meet the demand for their services. Finally, there were fewer studies of British programs, but initial reports suggested that hospice philosophy in England, as in the United States, had some influence on health care services as well as having been influenced by traditional health care services.

Hospice advocates avowed that integration with the NHS might lead to rapid spread of hospice services, but staff would be inadequately trained, hospice care would be subsumed by aggressive, cure-oriented treatments, and traditional hierarchical structures would be counterproductive to efforts by hospice staff to involve patients in decision making. As costs and the demand for services continued to rise, most programs sought partial reimbursement from the NHS, but they maintained administrative independence from the public health care system.

British physicians willingly referred terminally ill patients to hospice programs. British patients and families were also more interested in seeking hospice care because it gave them greater access to inpatient services (Kelly and Barber 1989). Research in the United Kingdom concurred with findings in the United States that being relieved of the stress of caregiving is an important need of families coping with a terminally ill relative.

> The rising proportion of deaths from cancer which now occur in hospitals and other institutions suggests that they are regarded as proper places in which to die, thus relieving families of some of the practical necessities associated with death. Any precise policy laid down as to where terminal care should take place would be doomed to failure from the outset. It is not only a matter of the patient's medical condition, but the patient's own circumstances and preferences will also have a profound influence." (Ford 1984, 210)

Evaluation of hospice programs was recommended, but British studies were even more limited than those in America. Only Saint Christopher's Hospice consistently studied the benefits of its services. Research assessing the quality of care among program types or the impact of hospice philosophy on families was inadequate. Those who did research outcomes found that pain control was more successful in hospices, that the hospice concept was acceptable to physicians and consumers, and that as hospice philosophy was integrated into acute health care systems it became more like mainstream medicine.

Although pain management was still most successful at Saint Christopher's and other independent facilities, pain management techniques developed by hospice physicians soon became accepted medical practices. Researchers at Saint Christopher's developed a drug mixture called Bromptom's Cocktail, a combination of heroin, cocaine, and alcohol, which was an effective treatment for the physical pain associated with terminal illnesses. Dying patients who received this treatment did not become addicted to the drug; by anticipating pain rather than treating it after it occurred drug doses were maintained below addictive levels. Listening to patients and addressing their emotional and spiritual pain were also part of pain management and symptom control. These latter aspects of pain control were often missing in hospice programs that were created as part of acute health care systems; these providers were less successful in reducing pain.

In contrast to most American hospice programs, British hospice programs often allowed nurses to control decisions about pain medication and fostered a more homelike environment. For example, less attention was paid to routines such as taking temperatures and pulses, even in hospital-based programs. Parkes and Parkes (1984) observed that patients at Saint Christopher's were more likely to feel they had access to staff who were available to provide them with support. A participant observation study of an NHS-sponsored program found that while initially this program was a "showcase" institution, as it slowly integrated with its sponsoring NHS hospital patients' emotional and spiritual needs became less well attended (Seale 1989).

When hospice care was integrated with acute care hospitals the impact of hospice philosophy was mixed. One study of an inpatient coronary care unit in a British general hospital found that it was possible to provide hospice-style care on this ward.

> Under conditions where nurses have the time to get to know dying patients, where nurses are assigned responsibility for the care of individual patients rather than just tasks, where a supportive and non-hierarchical relationship exists between staff, and when a policy of open disclosure of diagnosis and prognosis prevails, nursing care for the dying approaches the ideal of hospice care. (Seale 1989, 552)

Conversely, a survey of 98 hospice U.K. inpatient services where a medical director was present on the unit found that these providers were more likely to be identified as technically oriented and were more likely to use aggressive procedures such as blood transfusions or draining pleural effusions (Johnson, Rogers, Biswas, and Ahmedzai 1990).

**Canadian Programs** Canada's first hospice program, established in Montreal in 1975, was the Palliative Care Unit at the Royal Victoria Hospital, a teaching hospital affiliated with McGill University. As research on death and dying became common knowledge, certain staff members at the Royal Victoria Hospital recognized that they, too, paid insufficient attention to dying patients. Their desire to ameliorate these conditions was supported by the hospital's administration and board of directors. Although this hospice was developed in a fashion similar to that of many early American hospice programs, acquiring the approval of hospital administrators to get started was not as difficult as it was in America.

In 1973 a multidisciplinary team from the Royal Victoria's staff called the Ad Hoc Committee on Thanatology was formed to study the problem and make recommendations. The committee administered questionnaires to patients and medical staff to assess the emotional and physical needs of terminally ill patients and to assess medical staff's perceptions of them. According to the survey, patients wanted open and honest discussion of their situation, but professional staff resisted, ignored, or minimized dying patients' need to talk about their diagnosis and prognosis. These findings reinforced the committee's sentiment that services for the terminally ill were inadequate, and it recommended that a special hospital unit be created to resolve the problem. The hospital's administration readily accepted the recommendations and instituted plans to develop a hospice program.

The Palliative Care Unit functioned as a discrete entity within the acute care hospital. This model was later adopted by hospice groups in the United States. During its formative stage, program developers invited Elisabeth Kübler-Ross to lecture about death and dying, and members of the hospice team were sent to England to study at Saint Christopher's Hospice. Like British programs, the Palliative Care Unit allowed patients and families to decide whether they wanted to be in the hospital or at home.

This first Canadian program's design was a compromise between building a separate facility, which would have difficulty sustaining itself financially, and integrating the hospice concept with the acute health care system, which might impair the quality of services for both acutely ill and terminally ill patients. Hospice programs in Canada were not automatically supported by the government-sponsored national health insurance program, and obtaining funds to create independent facilities was therefore difficult.

The Ad Hoc Committee, however, did not want to integrate hospice care into hospital treatments. They asserted that the professional skills that enabled acute care staff to help patients "fight for life" were incompatible with the skills that allowed hospice staff to help patients and families "prepare for death" (Wilson, Ajemian, and Mount 1978). Consequently, it was decided that a separate unit with specially trained staff would better serve hospice patients. Since it first opened, the Palliative Care Unit has expanded to create a second unit and a home care service.

Initially, Canadian programs were almost exclusively created as special units in acute or chronic care hospitals. Only 42 percent of these programs were funded by the hospital's budget, thus allowing hospice directors to maintain control over their programs (Hudson 1990). As the concept of hospice care became more popular, however, volunteer groups began to imitate American hospice models, such as the case management or community-based program. As programs diversified they became essentially nursing services. The Hospice Care Program at Victoria General in Halifax is a case management model. Services are provided by a nurse with special training who interacts with terminally ill patients and with staff throughout the hospital, facilitating communication, spiritual support, and pain management. By 1986, of the 373 Canadian hospice programs, only 50 percent were affiliated with hospitals, and of those programs that were affiliated with hospitals 66 percent were consulting teams, not separate hospice units.

**Programs in Other Countries**  In West Germany hospice programs were introduced during the 1980s. The health care in this country is government funded, and although there are public, religious, and private hospitals, the services they provide are of a similar quality. According to Albrecht (1989), West German health care providers are ill equipped to deal with death and dying. Physicians are not trained in palliative care, and patients are likely to receive aggressive treatments up until the last minute of their lives. Moreover, legal restrictions on barbiturates prohibit prescribing these drugs around the clock, and physicians are reluctant to use barbiturates for pain management.

Another cultural distinction that made introducing hospice care to West Germans difficult is their attitude toward donating funds or time for health care services. West Germans are accustomed to supporting health care services through public revenues; fund-raising and volunteerism, common to program development in other countries, are little known practices.

Three inpatient units are now in place, and another 300 groups provide in-home hospice support to patients and families. Moreover, two organizations, Omega and German Hospice Aid, have been created to encourage support for hospice care and to develop interest in volunteerism.

The influence of the hospice movement has also been felt in countries that were previously dominated by communism. In 1971 the Catholic Church in Poland sponsored groups to discuss care of one's neighbor, particularly hospice care for the terminally ill. At first such groups were informal, volunteer attempts to develop hospice programs. Cicely Saunders visited Poland in 1978 to lecture about hospice care, and following her visit the Association of Friends of the Sick was organized. This group attempted to build a freestanding hospice in Krakow, but soon found that funding for a separate institution was unavailable. Instead the group developed a home care program that began providing services in 1981. By 1990, the concept of hospice care had become popular in Poland, and there were 20 programs in as many towns and cities. Home care services remained the dominant form, although a few programs were part of an inpatient hospital service (Sikorska 1991).

## Conclusion

Although falling short of its goal to create an autonomous form of care for the dying, the hospice movement continues to influence the nature of such care. Increased attention to pain control was facilitated by hospice activists, who brought new techniques to the attention of physicians. Moreover, the needs of special groups, such as AIDS patients and children suffering from cancer, renewed the purpose of the movement to alleviate the physical, emotional, and spiritual suffering of terminally ill people and their families.

*Chapter 9*

# Care of the Dying: A Persistent Social Issue

According to stage theory, social movements progress through five stages, the last being demise. Stage theorists anticipate that as a movement achieves political goals its momentum quickly dissipates. Typically, the deflection and co-optation processes reach a stage where the original efforts of the movement's participants are so diluted that the initial cause is all but forgotten; the original leaders are perceived as zealots and are withdrawn from positions of influence. Although the political course of the hospice movement has met with limited success, the movement has yet to reach a stage of demise because the issues that spurred its development remain potent. Western culture continues to be in conflict over the way people should die. This chapter briefly reviews the hospice movement's political struggle to achieve its ideals and the social forces that support continuing efforts to revolutionize care for the dying.

## The Struggle to Reform Terminal Care

The hospice movement's original intent was to establish an alternative method of care for the dying, but it cannot be said that this goal has or has not been achieved. Independence from the traditional medical care system is an important factor in whether or not a program can be considered an alternative. Insofar as hospice care providers offer palliative rather than aggressive services and encourage patients and families to take charge of treatment decisions, hospice is an alternative. Most hospice programs, however, have integrated with mainstream medicine and depend on it for referrals, making them more an extension of traditional health care service than a genuine alternative to it.

Early in the movement leaders chose to emphasize the importance of federal funding to support the movement's growth, and they failed to see the negative consequences of this decision. Moreover, as the movement progressed, many leaders seemed to forget that hospice was intended as a nontraditional approach to terminal care. "Its [the hospice movement's] founders were lay people. They were determined to treat the dying more humanely, and equally, to help society rethink the scope of 'medical' care. Yet, time and time again the various writers—all highly credentialed professionals—miss the opportunity to suggest that hospice represents a distinct philosophy and mission in caregiving that might change tradition rather than succumb to it" (Silver 1985, 10).

In forgetting the philosophy of the movement, leaders derailed it, preventing it from achieving its ideal goals. Despite avowals to be more accepting of the dying process, many hospice workers, like the rest of the population, were likely to want to avoid talking about death. During the early stages of program development, staff meetings encouraged open discussion about death. As programs proliferated such practices became less common.

A diminished concern for the social and psychological factors surrounding death was consistent with the drift away from a multidimensional approach to pain control. Hospice advocates were particularly attracted to the idea that there were ways to "cure" the physical pain of death, losing sight of the fact that pain control was a spiritual and emotional as well as physical process. Emphasizing the physical properties of death's pains and focusing on technological innovations marked a significant departure from the comprehensive approach to pain control favored by Cicely Saunders in England and emulated by early advocates of hospice care in the United States.

Finally, the tendency of movement participants to overstate and idealize their goals made reform of health care difficult. Skeptics viewed hospice advocates as morbid do-gooders and discounted the whole concept rather than appreciate its potential benefits. The concept of "good death" tended to idealize hospice care and set up unrealistic expectations about what providers of hospice care could accomplish (Liss-Levinson 1982; Mudd 1982). Perhaps what was lacking in many hospice programs was a mechanism for acknowledging that death was not pleasant, desirable, or good.

In hindsight, we can speculate about ways that the hospice movement's leaders might have better managed the movement's political course. Had they chosen to maintain purity of purpose in their efforts to assert patient and family control over treatment and therefore demedicalized the process, they might have established hospice centers with no ties to the acute health care system. But this was not what hospice advocates did, nor might such goals have been achievable. The movement represents a compromise of medicalizing and demedicalizing forces, and its experience in attempting to bring about change reflects an ongoing social struggle.

For example, during the past 20 years it has become common to attribute alcohol abuse to a disease process and to create medical treatments to cure those afflicted with it. Concomitantly, there has been a countertrend that attributes alcohol abuse to a moral failing, and stricter laws prosecuting offenders, along with nonmedical settings to reform problem drinkers, have been established. Neither method of constructing the problem ever succeeds in eliminating the other perspective, but rather each has its share of supporters who sustain their belief as to what causes and what stops alcohol abuse.

The hospice movement faced a similar dilemma in that the manner of death in this culture has been influenced by two opposing constructions. The first is the belief that acute health care has the capacity to overcome physical discomfort. The other is that death is a natural process and should be removed from mainstream medicine's influence. Each of these beliefs has merit, but determining when one or the other should take precedence is a difficult and often subjective process. Ongoing efforts to promote these perspectives help to perpetuate efforts to improve conditions, albeit in different ways, for the dying. Those who believe in the fight for life support scientific advances in treatment and are less concerned with questions of quality of life. In contrast, prolonging life often means protracted periods of pain, and no hope of meaningful life, therefore arousing social interest in ceasing treatment. The interplay of these medicalizing and demedicalizing forces has kept the hospice movement alive.

## The Persistence of the Hospice Movement

Activities by movement participants testify to the movement's persistence. Among these activities are leaders' continued involvement in the death with dignity movement, their continued belief in the hospice movement's original ideals, the development of new programs that reassert these ideals, and the social response to ethical dilemmas created by the ever-increasing sophistication of medical technology.

**Ties to the Death with Dignity Movement**  Initially, hospice advocates were among the participants of the death with dignity movement, but as the former group developed hospice programs and politicized the dying problem, they forged a separate social movement. The death with dignity movement never gained the momentum of the hospice movement, and its cause lost considerable popular appeal during the 1980s, but participants of the death with dignity movement have continued their efforts to alter attitudes toward death and dying.

The International Work Group on Death, Dying, and Bereavement continues to bring together advocates of death with dignity and advocates of hospice care. Although bereavement and spiritual services have not been adequately provided in hospice programs, work groups of the IWG persist in asserting their importance. Moreover, the IWG participates in helping new providers create hospice programs. One example is the IWG's work with the Omega Foundation, described below.

> The Omega Foundation comprises an interdisciplinary team, which provides palliative and bereavement care for dying patients and their families, both in their homes and in local hospitals. The team provides many lectures, and organizes seminars and conferences on the topics of death, dying, and bereavement with the aim of improving the quality of palliative care in Colombia. The IWG Board of Directors and its members strongly support the efforts of Dr. Isa de Jaramillo, the team, and the Board of Directors. The members of the IWG are willing to facilitate the further development of palliative care in Colombia through the Omega Foundation by serving as consultants and by providing reference materials and clinical experience. (*Death Studies* 1989, 319–20)

The international hospice movement has also made efforts to reduce resistance to the concept of hospice care. Among the problems that hospice advocates faced in this country were the lack of physician interest and of adequate research on the benefits of hospice care. In 1989 the International Hospice Institute was formed to conduct research and to give physicians opting to work in hospice programs credibility as specialists. As of 1990, about 500 physicians had become members (Magno 1990).

**The Enthusiasm of Movement Participants**  Leaders' optimism has been one of the movement's greatest assets. Rather than being daunted by political co-optations and deflections, many of the movement's early leaders still claim that hospice care is just beginning to exert its influence on American culture. They contend that emerging social issues will support their efforts to reform health care practices. The baby-boom generation, which has yet to reach the age when cancer is more likely to occur, the rising number of AIDS victims, and the increased demand for less costly health care services are among the factors that leaders claim will intensify the demand for humanistic approaches to caregiving, such as hospice care (Magno 1990; Stoddard 1991; Williams 1989).

Social movement theory suggests that as a movement's goals are compromised, idealists begin to be perceived as unrealistic and their influence diminishes. In the case of the hospice movement, although early leaders have been criticized by some, they still bring recruits to the hospice cause. Charismatic individuals such as Elisabeth Kübler-Ross and Cicely Saunders continue to attract new followers and to sustain the public's awareness of the plight of the dying.

Kübler-Ross lectures nationally about the need to discuss feelings about death and dying openly, and she conducts group and individual sessions to assist dying people in exploring their emotional and spiritual needs. She was also among the first to fight for humane services for AIDS patients. Saunders, who realized the hospice ideal at Saint Christopher's Hospice, has stated that the concept of hospice care had to continue to grow and change if it was to be a meaningful service. During the mid-1980s she observed that hospice programs had reached a point at which providers were prevented from helping dying patients by their own rules, "sacred cows" that inhibited creative and holistic practices. Saunders asserted, "If I could think of the most constructive thing to improve hospice it would be to go on a sacred cow shoot so that the field could go ahead" (Torrens 1985, 187).

**The Ongoing Development of New Programs**  Consumers have also played a part in the hospice movement's persistence. The increase of chronic debilitating conditions and the limited availability of acute care services have led more consumers to seek help in maintaining comfort and dignity during the last months of their lives, thus creating a demand for programs that offer holistic, noncure-oriented care, as originally intended by the hospice movement. Requests for hospice services by patients, families, and physicians have increased. Nationwide statistics on the use of the Medicare hospice benefit show that while only 2,000 beneficiaries elected to use it in 1984, 11,000 used it in 1986 (Davis 1988). Statistics at the state level indicate that use of hospice programs has also increased among those not eligible for Medicare. In Maine, for example, there are 20 hospice programs, a few of which are Medicare certified and only one of which has an inpatient unit, yet the demand for hospice care has doubled since 1986.

New programs that are similar to the early volunteer programs continue to be developed. These programs emphasize nonmedical, psychosocial support. One hospice program coordinator reported on a program begun in 1988 that was run primarily by volunteers. "We depend on our volunteers. We have wonderful volunteers, nurses, ministers, even physicians who are willing to do what they can to make people comfortable" (Siebold and Bucher 1990). To recruit volunteers this coordinator spoke at community group meetings about the services hospice care offered and the way that volunteers could make a difference to patients and families coping with terminal illness. Such new providers constitute the minority, but they preserve the hospice movement's original purpose.

**Ethical Dilemmas** Ethical issues surrounding the plight of the dying reinforce the need for the hospice movement. Two groups—those who want to allow death to occur naturally with minimal intervention and those who want to expedite death—continue to attract attention to the movement. The first group, potential consumers of hospice services, have been discussed above. Their increased number causes policymakers and physicians to look more favorably on alternatives, such as hospice programs. The second group, those who believe that death is preferable to suffering, help to raise support for hospice care indirectly.

"Assisted death" (a form of active euthanasia) is an unacceptable solution for the majority of Americans, but it continues to be proposed by a vocal minority. Although interest in assisted death does not directly create a demand for hospice care, it keeps the concept of hospice care as an alternative to assisted death before the public eye. Advocates assert that when methods of hospice care are employed properly, euthanasia is unnecessary. Robert Twycross, a physician and researcher at Saint Christopher's Hospice, purported:

I should stress that I am not in favour of "meddlesome" or "mindless" medical intervention at the end of life. I believe, for example, for an octogenarian to say "I've lived a good life and I am ready to go" is neither immoral nor anti-life. I still feel bound, however, by the cardinal medical ethical principal that I must achieve my treatment goal with the least risk to the patient's life. I have worked for nearly 20 years in palliative medicine/hospice care. During this time, my opinions on many issues both within and outwith clinical practice have changed. One that has not changed, however, is my belief that it would be a disaster for the medical profession to cross the Rubicon and to be permitted to use pharmacological means to precipitate death deliberately and specifically. (Twycross 1990, 796)

## Conclusion

The hospice movement has for most of its history been a study in contrasts. As easing death's pains became a goal of Western culture during the latter part of the twentieth century, social reformers emerged to ameliorate the dying problem. The beliefs that inspired the movement and the participants who espoused them were often in opposition. A demedicalized, humanistic approach to terminal care combined with a medicalized, treatment-oriented approach.

In the final analysis the plight of the dying continues to attract attention, albeit less now than during the 1960s and 1970s. What remains undefined is the construction of death in our culture. Is dying a medical event or an event in the life cycle? How one responds to this question influences who has control over the process—the individual or a medical technician. Given the increasing ability of medical practitioners to prolong life, this question will continue to be asked and collective endeavors organized to answer it.

# Appendix: Sources of Information on Hospice Care

The American Journal of Hospice Care
470 Boston Post Road
Weston, MA 02193

The Hospice Journal
75 Griswold Street
Binghamton, NY 13904

International Work Group on Death, Dying, and Bereavement
c/o Dr. John D. Morgan, Secretary
Kings College
266 Epworth Avenue
London, Ontario, CANADA N6A 2M3

National Hospice Organization
1901 North Fort Myer Drive, Suite 202
Arlington, VA 22209

Saint Christopher's Hospice
51–59 Lawrie Park Road
Sydenham, London, ENGLAND SE26 6DZ

Society for the Right to Die
250 West 57th Street
New York, NY 10107

# Notes

1. Other cultures also claim that hospitals have dehumanized death. According to Dracopoulis and Doxiades (1988), in Greece death traditionally was met with horror. Greeks did not romanticize the dying person, but openly grieved and expressed anger at the fact that life had ended. Contemporary urban Greek culture, however, has adopted Western medical technology, and dying people are more likely to be hospitalized. According to these researchers, this has led to death-denying practices similar to those observed in the United States. As in America, the dying are isolated from family and friends. The modern Greek may never witness the death of another human being unless he or she opts to be one of the specialists whose job it is to tend the sick.

2. In certain cultures, particularly less technologically advanced ones, active or passive euthanasia is common. Allowing children born with birth defects to starve to death, burying people alive when it is believed that they are dying, or, as in the case of the Eskimo, building the dying person an ice igloo as a sign of respect, have been accepted ways to deal with less functional members of society. This behavior is motivated by pragmatic need, not murderous desire. The Eskimos, for example, believed that they could not live in a house where someone had died, so placing the dying person in a separate igloo also insured against the loss of the family home during winter. A Luzon tribe in the Philippines also took a practical approach to the care of the sick. When someone was determined to be terminally ill, the tribe set aside a sum of money for his or her care. When the money was gone, they placed the dying person outside the hut on skins and assigned a child to sit with the ill person to swat flies and give him or her water until death occurred. These practices were celebrated by some form of feast or ceremonial ritual (Hefferman and Maynard 1977).

3. For instance, one policy developed by TEFRA was the DRGs (diagnosis related groups). DRGs, familiar to anyone who has required routine hospital care during the past 10 years, were an attempt by government policymakers to curb escalating hospital costs by restricting payments for routine procedures. The greatest problem resulting from such restrictions is that individual needs are not taken

into account. Payment is based on average length of stay, regardless of individual variations in healing. Consequently, discharge from hospitals is much quicker than it once was because when hospitals fail to meet length of stay restrictions they are forced to provide care without reimbursement.

4. As noted in chapter 7, findings on the effectiveness of pain management and symptom control techniques are mixed. Such ambiguity is a function of better knowledge about pain management techniques, but it also reflects poor training of hospice caregivers, particularly in community-based programs.

# Bibliography

Abdellah, F. G., B. C. Harper, and J. L. Lunceford. 1982. *Hospice Care in the United States: Information for Health Professionals and Health Care Providers*. Report. Baltimore: Health Care Financing Foundation, Subcommittee on Professional Education and Training Interagency Committee on New Therapies for Pain and Discomfort.

Abel, E. K. 1986. "The Hospice Movement: Institutionalizing Innovation." *International Journal of Health Services* 16 (1): 71–85.

Ackernecht, E. H. 1968. *A Short History of Medicine*. New York: Ronald Press.

Aiken, L. H. 1986. "Evaluation Research and Public Policy: Lessons from the NHS." *Journal of Chronic Diseases* 39: 1–4.

Aiken, L. H., and M. M. Marx. 1982. "Hospices: Perspectives on the Public Policy Debate." *American Psychologist* 37: 1271–79.

Albrecht, E. 1989. "The Development of Hospice Care in West Germany." *Journal of Palliative Care* 5 (3): 42–44.

Allen, N. 1990. "Hospice to Hospital in the Near East: Instance of Continuity and Change Late Antiquity." *Bulletin of History of Medicine* 64: 446–62.

Amenta, M. 1984. "Reimbursement Accreditation and the Movement's Future." *American Journal of Hospice Care* (Winter) 10–14.

———. 1988. "Nurses as Primary Spiritual Care Workers." *The Hospice Journal* 4 (3): 47–56.

Ariès, P. 1974. *Western Attitudes toward Death: From the Middle Ages to the Present*. Baltimore: Johns Hopkins University Press.

Back, K. 1989. *Family Planning and Population Control*. Boston: Twayne Publishers.

Bass, D. 1985. "The Hospice Ideology and Success of Hospice Care." *Research on Aging* 7 (3): 307–27.

Beavan, J. 1959. "Euthanasia." *New York Times*, 9 August.

Beckwith, B. E., J. E. Beckwith, T. L. Gray, et al. 1990. "Identification of Spouses at High Risk during Bereavement." *Hospice Journal* 6 (3): 7–8.

Benoliel, J. Q. 1979. "Dying in an Institution." In *Dying Facing the Facts*, edited by H. Wass. New York: McGraw-Hill.

Blauner, R. 1966. "Death and Social Structures." *Psychiatry* 29: 379.

Boffey, R. M. 1987. "Report to Congress Terms Gains on Cancer Overstated Since 1950." *New York Times*, 16 April.

Breindel, L., and R. Boyle. 1979. "Implementing a Multiphased Hospice Program." *Hospital Progress* 3: 42–45.

Bronowski, J. 1973. *The Ascent of Man*. London: British Broadcasting Corp.

Buckingham, R. W. 1983. *The Complete Hospice Guide*. New York: Harper and Row.

_____. 1982–83. "Hospice Care in the United States: The Process Begins." *Omega* 13 (2): 159–71.

Buckingham, R. W., S. A. Lack, B. M. Mount, L. D. MacLean, and J. T. Collins. 1976. "Living with the Dying: Use of the Technique of Participant Observation." *Canadian Medical Association Journal* 115: 1211–15.

Buckingham, R. W., and L. Loveday. 1983. "Hospice Programs and Dying Children." In *The Complete Hospice Guide*, edited by R. W. Buckingham. New York: Harper and Row.

Buckingham, R. W., and D. Lupu. 1982. "A Comparative Study of Hospice Services in the United States." *American Journal of Public Health* 72 (5): 455–62.

Bulkin, W., and H. Lukashok. 1988. "RX for Dying: The Case for Hospice." *New England Journal of Medicine* 318 (6): 376–78.

Bullough, V., and B. Bullough. 1972. "A Brief History of Medical Practice." In *Medical Men and Their Work*, edited by E. Freidson and J. Lorber. Chicago: Aldine Press.

Butler, R. 1979. "The Need for Quality Hospice Care." *QRB* 5 (5): 2–8.

Butterfield-Picard, H., and J. B. Magno. 1982. "Hospice the Adjective, Not the Noun: The Future of a National Priority." *American Psychologist* 37: 1254–59.

Byrd, S., and K. Taylor. 1989. "Evaluating Hospice Care: A Practical Approach." *American Journal of Hospice Care* 6 (1): 41–46.

Callahan, D. 1979. Letter from the Director. *Hastings Center Report*. 9 (1): 1.

Caplan, G. 1964. *Principles of Preventive Psychiatry*. New York: Basic Books.

Carey, D. A. 1986. *Hospice Inpatient Environments: Compenduim and Guidelines*. New York: Van Nostrand Reinhold Co.

Carney, K., B. Borbst, and B. Burns. 1989. "The Impact of Reimbursement: The Case of Hospice." *Hospice Journal* 5 (3–4): 73–91.

Carwein, V., and C. Longley. 1989. "Aids Dementia: Assessment and Interventions for Home Hospice Care." *Caring*, June, 21–24.

Cassileth, B. R., C. Brown, C. Lavierte, et al. 1989. "Medical Students' Reactions to a Hospice Preceptorship." *Journal Cancer Education* 4 (4): 261–63.

Castiglione, A. 1947. *A History of Medicine*. New York: Alfred A. Knopf.

Chapman, J., and J. Goodall. 1979. "Dying Children Need Help Too." *British Medical Journal* 1: 593–94.

Cherry, L. 1982. "Hospice: New Help for the Dying." *Glamour*, March, 256–57, 309–14.

Cimino, J. E. 1983. "Caring for the Terminally Ill: The Story of an American Hospital." In *Hospice: U.S.A.*, edited by A. Kutscher et al. New York: Columbia University Press.

Cody, P., and N. Naierman. 1990. "Evaluation of the Cost Effectiveness of a Collaborative Liaison Program." *Hospice Journal* 6 (3): 47–61.

Cohen, K. 1979. *Hospice: Prescription for Terminal Care*. Germantown, Md.: Aspen Systems Corp.

Connor, S. R., and L. K. Kraymer. 1982. "The Evolution of an Urban Based Hospice Program." *Family and Community Health* 5 (3): 39–53.

Conrad, P., and J. W. Schneider. 1980. *Deviance and Medicalization, from Badness Sickness*. Saint Louis: Mosby Press.

Coordinating Council for Independent Living. 1986. "Hospice State of the Art." Morgantown, W.V.: Council Report.

Corbett, T. L., and D. M. Hai. 1979. "Searching for Euthanatos: The Hospice Alternative." *Hospital Progress* 60 (March): 38–41.

Corless, I. B. 1983. "The Hospice Movement in North America." In *Hospice Principles of Practice*, edited by C. Corr and D. Corr. New York: Springer Publication Co.

_____. 1985. "Implications of the New Hospice Legislation and the Accompanying Regulations." *Nursing Clinics of North America* 20 (2): 281–98.

Corr, C., and D. Corr. 1983. *Hospice Principles of Practice*. New York: Springer Publication Co.

Creek, L. V. 1982. "A Homecare Hospice Profile: Description, Evaluation, and Cost Analysis." *Journal of Family Practice* 14 (1): 53–58.

Crowther, C. E. 1980. "The Stalled Hospice Movement." *The New Physician* 29: 26–28.

Dailey, A. A. 1988. "About Our Children." *American Journal of Hospice Care* 5 (1): 15–16.

Dailey, A. A., and S. DiTullio. 1988. "Melinda House." *American Journal of Hospice Care* 5 (5): 13–15.

Davidson, G. 1978. *The Hospice Development and Administration*. Washington, D.C.: Hemisphere Publishing Corp.

Davidson, J. 1990. "AIDS Hospice." *Interior Design* 61 (5): 204–5.

Davis, F. A. 1988. "Medicare Hospice Benefit: Early Program Experience." *Health Care Financing Review* 9 (4): 99–111.

*Death Studies*. 1989. "Statement of Support for the Omega Foundation in Colombia from the International Work Group on Death, Dying, and Bereavement." 13: 319–322.

Dempsey, D. 1975. *The Way We Die: An Investigation of Death and Dying in America Today*. New York: McGraw-Hill.

De Souza, L. J. 1981. "Asia." In *Hospice: The Living Ideal*, edited by C. Saunders et al. London: Edward Arnold.

Dobihal, E. F. 1974. "Talk or Terminal Care." *Connecticut Medicine* 38 (July): 364–67.

Dooley, J. 1982. "The Corruption of Hospice." *Public Welfare* 40 (Spring): 35–41.

Downie, P. A. 1973. "Havens of Peace." *Nursing Times* 69 (33): 1068–70.

Dracopoulis, S., and S. Doxiades. 1988. "In Greece Lament for the Dead, Denial of Dying." *Hastings Center Report*, August supplement, 15–18.

DuBois, P. 1980. *The Hospice Way of Death*. New York: Human Science Press.

Dubos, R. J. 1959. *Mirage of Health: Utopias, Progress, and Biological Change*. New York: Anchor Books.

DuBoulay, S. 1984. *Cicely Saunders, Founder of the Modern Hospice Movement*. London: Hodder and Staughton.

Dunkin, A., ed. 1990. "Living Wills: In Defense of Your Right to Die." *Business Week*, 30 July, 78–79.

Dunnet, S. 1973. "I Know I'm Dying." *New York Times*, 25 November.

Durkheim, E. 1947. *Division of Labor*. Translated by G. Simpson, Glencoe, Ill.: Free Press.

Dush, D. M. 1988. "Trends in Hospice Research and Psychosocial Palliative Care." *Hospice Journal* 4 (3): 13–28.

Edmondson, B. 1990. "AIDS and Aging." *American Demographics* 12 (3): 28–31.

Eissler, K. 1955. *The Psychiatrist and the Dying Patient*. New York: International University Press.

Enck, R. E. 1986. "Hospice: The Game Is Not Over." *Seminars in Oncology* 13 (1): 128–29.

Epstein, S. 1978. *The Politics of Cancer*. Sierra Club Books: San Francisco.

Ewens, J., and P. Herrington. 1983. *Hospice: A Handbook for Families and Others Facing Terminal Illness*. Santa Fe, N.M.: Bear and Company.

Falk, R. H. 1984. "The Death of Death with Dignity." *American Journal of Medicine* 77: 775–76.

Farrow, G. 1981. "Helen House: Our First Hospice for Children." *Nursing Times,* 12 August, 1433–34.

Faulkner, H. P., and D. Kugler. 1981. *JCAH Hospice Project Interim Report Phase I.* Chicago.

Feifel, H. 1959. *The Meaning of Death.* New York: Human Science Press.

_____. 1977a. *New Meanings of Death.* New York: McGraw-Hill.

_____. 1977b. "Death and Dying in Modern America." *Death Education* 1: 5–14.

Fennel, M. L., and R. B. Werneeke. 1988. *The Diffusion of Medical Innovations: An Applied Network Analysis.* New York: Plenum Press.

Fisher, D. H. 1978. *Growing Old in America.* London: Oxford University.

Foley, K. M. 1989. "Controversies in Cancer Pain." *Cancer* 63 (11): 2257–65.

Ford, G. 1984. "Terminal Care in the National Health Service." In *The Management of Terminal Malignant Disease,* 2d ed., edited by C. Saunders. London: Edward Arnold.

Foster, Z. 1979. "Standards of Hospice Care: Assumptions and Principles." *Health and Social Work* 4: 118–28.

Foster Z., F. Wald, and H. J. Wald. 1978. "The Hospice Movement: A Backward Glance at its First Two Decades." Author's reprint.

Fox, R. 1974. *Experiment Perilous: Physicians and Patients Facing the Unknown.* Philadelphia: University of Pennsylvania Press.

_____. 1979. *Essays in Medical Sociology.* New York: John Wiley and Sons.

_____. 1980. *The Social Meaning of Death.* Philadelphia: American Academy of Political and Social Science.

_____. 1989. *The Sociology of Medicine.* Englewood Cliffs, N.J.: Prentice-Hall.

Frankl, V. 1963. *Man's Search for Meaning.* New York: Washington Press.

Freidson, E. 1970a. *Medical Dominance.* New York: Atherton Press.

_____. 1970b. *Profession of Medicine.* New York: Dodd, Mead and Co.

_____. 1985. "The Reorganization of the Medical Profession." *Medical Care Review* 42 (1): 11–34.

Fryer, J. 1982. "The International Work Group of Death, Dying, and Bereavement." Unpublished report.

Fulton, R. 1977. "The Sociology of Death." *Death Education* 1: 15–25.

Fulton, R., and G. Owen. 1981. "Hospice in America." In *Hospice: The Living Ideal,* edited by C. Saunders et al. London: Edward Arnold.

Galazka, M. 1990. "Can Hospice Rehabilitate Offenders?" *American Journal of Hospice Care* 7 (1): 17–18.

Garrison, F. 1929. *History of Medicine*. Philadelphia: W. B. Saunders and Co.

General Accounting Office. 1979. *Hospice Care: A Growing Concept in the United States, Report to Congress*. Washington, D.C.

_____. 1989. "Medicare Program Provisions and Payments Discourage Hospice Participation." Washington, D. C.

Giacquinta, B. 1989. "Researching the Effects of AIDS on Families." *American Journal of Hospice Care* 6 (3): 31–36.

Gilmore, A. 1989. "Hospice Development in the United Kingdom." In *Encyclopedia of Death*, edited by R. J. Kastenbaum and B. K. Kastenbaum. Phoenix: Oryx Press.

Gochman, D. S., and G. S. Bonham. 1988. "Physicians and the Hospice Decision: Awareness, Discussion, Reasons, Satisfaction." *Hospice Journal* 4 (1): 25–53.

Glaser, B., and A. L. Strauss. 1965. *Awareness of Dying*. Chicago: Aldine Press.

Gotay, C. C. 1983. "Models of Terminal Care." *Clinical and Investigative Medicine* 6: 131–41.

Gray-Toft, P., and J. G. Anderson. 1983. "Hospice Care: A Better Way of Caring for the Living." In *Hospice: U.S.A.*, edited by A. H. Kutscher et al. New York: Columbia University Press.

Greer, D. 1985. "Hospice: From Social Movement to Health Care Industry." *Transactions of American Clinical Climatological Association* 97: 82–7.

Greer, D., and V. Mor. 1985. "How Medicare Is Altering the Hospice Movement." *Hastings Center Report* 15: 5–9.

Greer, D., V. Mor, J. N. Morris, S. Sherwood, D. Kidder, and H. Birnbaum. 1986. "An Alternative in Terminal Care: Results of the National Hospice Study." *Journal of Chronic Disease* 39 (1): 9–26.

Guenette, H. 1989. "The Legacy of Rose Hawthorne." *Shore* (Winter): 24–26.

Hackley, J. 1979. "Financing and Accrediting Hospices." *Hospital Progress* 60: 51–53.

Halper, T. 1987. "Life and Death in a Welfare State: End-stage Renal Disease in the United Kingdom." In *Dominant Issues in Medical Sociology*, edited by H. Schwartz. New York: Random House.

Hamilton, M., and H. Reid. 1980. *A Hospice Handbook: A New Way to Care for the Dying*. Grand Rapids, Mich.: William B. Eerdmans Publishing Co.

Hannon, E. L., and J. F. O'Donnell. 1984. "An Evaluation of Hospices in the New York State Demonstration Project." *Inquiry* 21 (Winter): 338–48.

Hare, J. E. 1983. "The Hospice Movement and the Acceptance of Death." In *Hospice: U.S.A.*, edited by A. H. Kutscher et al. New York: Columbia University Press.

Hays, R. D., and S. Arnold. 1986. "Patient and Family Satisfaction with Care for the Terminally Ill." *Hospice Journal* 2 (3): 129–50.

Hefferman, R., and C. Maynard. 1977. "Living and Dying with Dignity: The Rise of Old Age and Dying as Social Problems." In *This Land of Promises: The Rise and Fall of Social Problems in America*, edited by A. Mauss and J. Wolfe. New York: J. B. Lippincott Co.

Hinton, J. 1977. *Dying*. Harmondsworth, England: Penguin Books.

Holden, C. 1978. "Hospice: For the Dying, Relief from Pain and Fear." *Science* 193 (4251): 389-91.

Hospice, Inc. 1974. Newsletter. December.

———. 1975. *Hospice*, March.

———. 1976. *Hospice*, April–June.

———. 1978. *Hospice*, June.

Houts, P., J. M. Yasko, H. A. Harvey, S. B. Kahn, et al. 1988. "Unmet Needs of Persons with Cancer in Pennsylvania during the Period of Terminal Care." *Cancer* 62: 627–34.

Hoyer, R. G. 1990. "Public Policy and the American Hospice Movement: The Tie That Binds." *Caring* 9 (3): 30–35.

Hudson, J. E. 1990. "Profile of Canadian Hospital-Based Palliative Care." *American Journal of Hospice and Palliative Care* 7 (3): 35–41.

Humphry, D. 1991. *Final Exit: The Practicalities of Self-Deliverance and Assisted Suicide for the Dying*. Los Angeles: Hemlock Society.

———. 1984. *Let Me Die before I Wake*. Los Angeles: Hemlock Society.

Humphry, D., and A. Wickett. 1986. *The Right to Die: Understanding Euthanasia*. New York: Harper and Row.

Illich, I. 1976. *Medical Nemesis: The Exploration of Health*. New York: Pantheon Books.

International Work Group on Death, Dying, and Bereavement. 1979. "Assumptions and Principles Underlying Standards for Terminal Care." *American Journal of Nursing*, February, 296–97.

Jenkins, L., and A. C. Cook. 1981. "The Rural Hospice: Integrating Formal and Informal Helping Systems." *Social Work* 25 (5): 414–16.

Johnson, I. S., C. Rogers, B. Biswas, and S. Ahmedzai. 1990. "What Do Hospices Do? A Survey of Hospices in the United Kingdom and Republic of Ireland." *British Medical Journal* 6727 (300): 791–92.

Jones, P. 1988. "How Has the Medicare Benefit Changed Hospice?" *Caring* 7 (8): 8–11.

Kane, R. L. 1986. "Lessons from Hospice Evaluations." *Hospice Journal* 2 (3): 3–8.

Kane, R. L., J. Wales, L. Bernstein, A. Leibowitz, and S. Kaplan. 1984. "A Randomized Controlled Trial of Hospice Care." *Lancet* 1: 890–94.

Kass, L. R. 1975. "Regarding the End of Medicine and the Pursuit of Health." *Public Interest* 40 (Summer): 11–42.

Kastenbaum, R. J. 1978. "Death, Dying, and Bereavement in Old Age." *Aged Care and Services Review* 1: 200–207.

_____. 1989. *Encyclopedia of Death*. Phoenix: Onyx Press.

_____. 1991. *Death, Society, and Human Experience*. New York: Macmillan Publishing Co.

Kastenbaum, R. J., and P. T. Costa. 1977. "Psychological Perspectives on Death." *Annual Review of Psychology* 28: 225–49.

Keller, C. P., and H. R. Bell. 1984. "The New Hospice Medicare Benefit." *Post Graduate Medicine* 75 (2): 71–73.

Kelly, M., and H. Barber. 1989. "Comparing Rural and Urban Hospices." *Practitioner* 233 (1473): 1063–65.

Kerbo, H. 1982. "Movements of Crises and Movements of Affluence." *Journal of Conflict Resolution* 26 (4): 645–63.

Kidder, D. 1987. *Health Care Financing: Medicare Hospice Benefit Program Evaluation*. Baltimore: U.S. Department of Health and Human Services.

Klagsbrun, S. 1982. "Ethics in Hospice Care." *American Psychologist* 37: 1263–65.

_____. 1983. "The Politics of Expanding Hospice Care." In *Hospice: U.S.A.*, edited by A. H. Kutscher et al. New York: Columbia University Press.

Klandermans, B., H. Kriesi, and S. Tarrow, eds. 1988. *International Social Movement Research Vol. 1*. Greenwich, Conn.: JAI Press.

Klandermans, B., and S. Tarrow. 1988. "Mobilization into Social Movements." In *International Movement Research*, edited by B. Klandermans, et al. Greenwich, Conn.: JAI Press.

Knight, C. F. 1990. "Networking with the Gay Community to Meet the Needs of AIDS Patients: Special Considerations for Volunteer Training." *American Journal of Hospice Care* 7 (1): 31–35.

Koff, T. 1980. *Hospice, A Caring Community*. Cambridge, Mass.: Winthrop Publishers.

Kohut, J., and S. Kohut. 1984. *Hospice, Caring for the Terminally Ill*. Springfield, Ill.: Charles C. Thomas Publishing.

Korhman, A. F. 1985. "Commentary: Physicians' Attitudes toward Hospice Care." In *Quality Care for the Terminally Ill*, edited by K. Gardiner. Chicago: JCAH.

Kramer, L. 1989. *Reports from the Holocaust—The Making of an AIDS Activist*. New York: St. Martin's Press.

Krant, M. J. 1974. *Dying and Dignity: The Meaning and Control of a Personal Death.* Springfield, Ill. Charles C. Thomas Publishing.

_____. 1978. "Sounding Board: The Hospice Movement." *New England Journal of Medicine* 299: 546–49.

Krant, M. J., M. Beiser, G. Adler, and L. Johnson. 1976. "The Role of a Hospital-based Psychosocial Unit in Terminal Cancer Illness and Bereavement." *Journal of Chronic Disease* 29: 115–27.

Kriebel, M. 1989. "A Profile of Hospice Programs in Pennsylvania." *Hospital Journal* 5 (3–4): 51–71.

Kriesi, H. 1989. "New Social Movement and the New Class in the Netherlands." *AJS* 98 (4): 1078–116.

Krikorian, D. A., and D. H. Moser. 1985. "Satisfaction and Stresses Experienced by Professional Nurses in Hospice Programs." *American Journal of Hospice Care* 2 (1): 25–33.

Kübler-Ross, E. 1969. *On Death and Dying.* New York: MacMillan.

Kulys, R., and M. A. Davis, Sr. 1986. "An Analysis of Social Services in Hospices." *Social Work* 31(6): 448–56.

Kutscher, A. H. 1983. *Hospice: U.S.A.* New York: Columbia University Press.

Kutzen, H. S. 1986. "A Community Approach to AIDS through Hospice: Louisiana Program Promotes High Quality of Life." *American Journal of Hospice Care*, March-April, 17–23.

Lack, S., and R. W. Buckingham. 1978. *The First American Hospice: Three Years of Home Care.* New Haven, Conn.: Hospice, Inc.

Labierte, L., and V. Mor. 1988. "The Hospice Volunteer." In *The Hospice Experiment*, edited by V. Mor et al. Baltimore: Johns Hopkins University Press.

Lamers, W. M. 1978. "Marin County Development of a Hospice Program." *Death Education* 2: 53–62.

_____. 1988. "Hospice Research: Some Reflections." *The Hospice Journal* 4 (3): 3–12.

Lamerton, R. 1975. "The Need for Hospices." *Nursing Times* 71: 154–57.

Landis, J. R. 1980. *Sociology: Concepts and Characteristics.* 4th ed. Belmont, Calif.: Wadsworth Publishing Co.

Lattanzi-Licht, M. E. 1989. "Bereavement Services: Practice and Problems." *Hospital Journal* 5 (1): 1–28.

Lautner, H., and J. Meyer. 1984. "Active Euthanasia without Consent—Historical Comment on a Current Debate." *Death Studies* 8 (2): 89–98.

Lentz, R. J., and L. J. Ramsey. 1988. "The Psychologist Consultant on the Hospice Team: One Example of the Model." *Hospice Journal* 4 (2): 55–63.

Lerman, D. 1988. "Hospital-Hospice Survey." *American Journal of Hospice Care* 5 (1): 28–31.

Lescohier, D. 1990. "Hospice Care for Minorities." *American Journal of Hospice and Palliative Care* 7 (5): 10.

Liegner, L. M. 1975. "Saint Christopher's Hospice, 1974: Care of the Dying Patient." *JAMA* 234: 1047–48.

Liss-Levinson, W. S. 1982. "Reality Perspectives for Psychological Services in a Hospice Program." *American Psychologist 37*: 1266–70.

_____. 1983. "A Comprehensive Geriatric Center." In *Hospice: U.S.A.*, edited by A. Kutscher et al. New York: Columbia University Press.

Lofland, L. 1975. *Toward a Theory of Death and Dying*. Beverly Hills: Sage Publications.

_____. 1978. *The Craft of Dying*. Beverly Hills: Sage Publications.

Lorber, J. 1981. "Physicians and Everyone Else: The Structure of the Modern Medical Profession." Unpublished paper.

Lynn, J. 1985. "Ethics in Hospice Care." In *Hospice Handbook: A Guide For Managers and Planners*, edited by L. F. Paradis. Rockville, Md.: Aspen Systems Corp.

McCann, B. 1982. "Project Update." *NHO President's Letter*, October.

_____. 1985. *Hospice Project Report*. Chicago: JCAH.

_____. 1988. Preface. In *The Hospice Experiment*, edited by V. Mor et al. Baltimore: Johns Hopkins University Press.

McCarthy, J., and M. Zald. 1973. *Social Movements in an Organization Society*. New Brunswick, N.J.: General Learning Press.

_____. 1979. *The Dynamics of Social Movements*. Cambridge, Mass.: Winthrop Publishers.

McCusker, J. 1984. "Development of Scales to Measure Satisfaction and Preferences Regarding Long Term and Terminal Care." *Medical Care* 22 (5): 476–93.

MacDonald, D. 1989. "Non-admissions: The Other Side of the Hospice Story." *American Journal of Hospice Care* 6 (2): 17–19.

McDuff, H. C., M. E. Toms, J. Gordon, and D. Rehm. 1990. "AIDS and Hospice Care of Rhode Island." *Rhode Island Medical Journal* 73 (July): 303.

MacEachern, M. T. 1957. *Hospital Organization and Management*. Chicago: Physician's Record Co.

McNulty, E. G., and R. A. Holderby. 1983. *Hospice: A Caring Challenge*. Springfield, Ill.: Charles C. Thomas Publishing.

Maddison, D., and W. L. Walker. 1967. "Factors Affecting the Outcome of Conjugal Bereavement." *British Journal of Psychiatry* 113: 1057–67.

Magno, J. B. 1990. "The Hospice Concept of Care: Facing the 1990s." *Death Studies* 14: 109–19.

Malcom, A. H. 1990. "Nancy Cruzan: End to Long Goodbye." *New York Times*, 29 December.

Marcuse, H. 1959. "The Ideology of Death." In *The Meaning of Death*, edited by H. Feifel. New York: McGraw-Hill.

Martin, J. P. 1986. "The AIDS Home Care and Hospice Program: A Multidisciplinary Approach to Caring for Persons with AIDS." *American Journal of Hospice Care* 3 (2): 35–37.

Mauss, A. 1975. *Social Problems as Social Movements*. New York: J. B. Lippincott Co.

Mechanic, D. 1968. *Medical Sociology: A Selective View*. New York: Free Press.

Meyers, H. I. 1990. "Minorities and Hospice Care." *American Journal of Hospice Care* 6 (4): 18–22.

Miller, S. M. 1971. *Max Weber*. New York: Thomas Y. Cromwell Co.

Millett, N. 1979. "Challenging Society's Approach to Death." *Health and Social Work* 4 (1): 117–28.

Millison, M. B., and J. R. Dudley. 1990. "The Importance of Spirituality in Hospice Work." *Hospice Journal* 6 (3): 63–78.

Mitford, J. 1963. *The American Way of Death*. New York: Simon and Schuster.

Moinpour, C. M., L. Polisar, and D. A. Conrad. 1990. "Factors Associated with Length of Stay in Hospice." *Medical Care* 28 (4): 363–8.

Monroe, M. 1973. *A Practical Guide to Long Term Care and Health Administration*. Greenville, N.Y.: Panel Publishing.

Mor, V. 1985. "Commentary: Results of Hospice Evaluations—A View from the N.H.S." In *Quality Care for the Terminally Ill*, edited by K. Gardiner. Chicago: JCAH.

_____. 1987. *Hospice Care Systems: Structure, Process, Costs, and Outcomes*. New York: Springer Publication Co.

Mor, V., D. Greer, and R. Kastenbaum. 1988. *The Hospice Experiment*. Baltimore: Johns Hopkins University Press.

Mor, V., and J. Hiris. 1983. "Determinants of Site of Death among Hospice Care Patients." *Journal of Health and Social Behavior* 24: 375–85.

Mount, B. 1985. "Four Clinical Areas That Confront and Challenge Hospice Professionals." *American Journal of Hospice Care* 2 (6): 22–29.

Mudd, P. 1982. "High Ideals and Hard Cases: The Evolution of a Hospice." *Hastings Center Report* 12 (2): 11–14.

Munley, A. 1983. *The Hospice Alternative: A New Context for Death and Dying*. New York: McGraw-Hill.

National Conference on Social Welfare. 1978. *The Hospice as a Social Institution*. Report of the Pre-Forum Institute of the 105th Annual Forum of the National Conference on Social Welfare, Los Angeles.

National Hospice Organization. 1979. *Delivery and Payment of Hospice Services: Investigative Study*. Arlington, Va.

―――. 1985. *Hospice: A Model Benefit*. Arlington, Va.

Neigh, J. E. 1990. "How Hospices Finally Got a Rate Increase." *American Journal of Hospice and Palliative Care* 7 (2): 14–9.

Nettler, G. 1967. "Review Essay: On Death and Dying." *Social Problems* 14 (3): 335–43.

Neubauer, B. V., and C. L. Hamilton. 1990. "Racial Differences in Attitudes toward Hospice Care." *Hospice Journal* 6 (1): 37–48.

*New York State Journal of Medicine.* 1989. "Designated Care Programs for Patients with AIDS and HIV Related Illnesses in Designated Care Centers." September, 542–43.

Ogg, E. 1959. *When a Family Faces Cancer*. New York: Public Affairs Pamphlets.

―――. 1985. *Facing Death and Loss*. Lancaster, Pa.: Technomic Publishing Company.

Olson, M. 1965. *The Logic of Collective Action: Public Goods and the Theory of Groups*. Cambridge, Mass.: Harvard University Press.

Osterweiss, M., and D. S. Champagne. 1979. "The U.S. Hospice Movement: Issues in Development." *American Journal of Public Health* 69: 492–96.

Paloma, M. 1982. *The Charismatic Movement*. Boston: Twayne Publishers.

Paradis, L. F. 1988. "An Assessment of Sociology's Contribution to Hospice: Priorities of Future Research." *Hospice Journal* 4 (3): 57–72.

Paradis, L. F., and S. B. Cummings. 1986. "The Evolution of Hospice in America toward Organizational Homogeneity." *Journal of Health and Social Behavior* 27: 370–86.

Parkes, C. M. 1979. "Terminal Care: Evaluation of Inpatient Service at Saint Christopher's Hospice, Part I and Part II. Self-Assessment of Effects of the Service on the Patient." *Postgraduate Medical Journal* 55: 517–27.

Parkes, C.M., B. Benjamin, and R. G. Fitzgerald. 1969. "Broken Heart: A Statistical Study of Increased Mortality among Widowers." *British Medical Journal* 1 (March): 740–43.

Parkes, C. M., and J. Parkes. 1984. "Hospice versus Hospital Care." *Post Graduate Medicine* 60: 120–24.

Parry, J. 1983. "Social Work Satisfaction in Relation to the Ideal Model of Care." Ph.D. diss., Wurzweiller School of Social Work.

Parsons, T. 1972. "Definitions of Illness and Health in Light of American Values and Social Structure." In *Patients, Physicians and Illness*, edited by E. G. Jaco. New York: Free Press.

Pawling-Kaplan, M., and P. O'Connor. 1989. "Hospice Care for Minorities: An Analysis of a Hospital-Based Inner City Palliative Care Service." *American Journal of Hospice Care* 6 (4): 13–20.

Peele, S. 1989. *Diseasing of America.* Lexington, Mass.: Lexington Books.

Perrollaz, L., and M. Mollica. 1981. "Public Knowledge of Hospice Care." *Nursing Outlook* 29: 46–48.

Phillips, C. 1991. "Lifeline to Hope." *Reader's Digest*, April, 37–44.

Randolph, J. 1982. "A Federal Role in Hospice Care?" *American Psychologist* 37: 1249–53.

Relman, A. 1987. "The New Medical-Industrial Complex." In *Dominant Issues in Medical Sociology*, edited by H. Schwartz. New York: Random House.

Rhymes, J. 1990. "Hospice Care in America." *JAMA* 264 (3): 369–72.

Richman, J. M., and L. B. Rosenfeld. 1988. "Demographic Profile of Individuals with Knowledge of Hospice." *American Journal of Hospice Care* 5 (1): 36–39.

Rinaldi, A., and M. C. Kearl. 1990. "The Hospice Farewell: Ideological Perspectives of Its Professional Practitioners." *Omega* 21 (4): 283–300.

Ritzer, G., and Walczak, D. 1986. *Working: Conflict and Change.* Englewood Cliffs, N.J.: Prentice-Hall.

Rohrschneider, R. 1990. "The Roots of Public Opinion toward New Social Movements." *American Journal of Political Science* 34 (1): 1–30.

Rosen, G. 1963. "The Hospital, Historical Sociology." In *The Hospital in Modern Society*, edited by E. Freidson. New York: Free Press.

Rossman, P. 1977. *Hospice.* New York: Fawcett Columbine.

Russell, G. M. 1985. "Hospice Programs and the Hospice Movement: An Investigation Based on the General Systems Theory." Ph.D. diss., Graduate School of the University of Colorado.

Sack, K. 1989. "Bronx Hospice, Facing a Chronic Deficit, to Close." *New York Times*, 23 November.

Saunders, C. M. 1976. "The Problem of Euthanasia." *Nursing Times* 55: 960–61.

_____. 1976. "Care of the Dying." *Nursing Times*, July.

_____. 1978. "Appropriate Treatment, Appropriate Death." In *The Management of Terminal Disease*, edited by C. Saunders. London: Edward Arnold.

_____. 1981a. *Hospice: The Living Ideal.* Philadelphia: W. B. Saunders Co.

_____. 1981b. Preface. In *Hospice Complete Care for the Terminally Ill*, edited by J. M. Zimmerman. Baltimore: Urban and Schwartzenberg.

_____. 1987. "Hospice for AIDS Patients." *American Journal of Hospice Care* 4 (6): 7.

Scarborough, J. 1969. *Roman Medicine*. New York: Cornell University Press.

Schnaper, N., and P. Wiernick. 1983. "The Hospice: New Wine in Old Bottles." *Maryland State Medical Journal* (February): 102–5.

Schneidman, E. 1973. *Deaths of Man*. New York: New York Times Book Co.

Schoenberg, B., A. C. Carr, D. Peretz, and A. H. Kutscher. 1974. *Anticipatory Grief*. New York: Columbia University Press.

Seale, Clive F. 1989. "What Happens in Hospices: A Review of Research Evidence." *Social Science and Medicine* 28 (6): 551–59.

Sedgwick, P. 1982. *Psycho-Politics*. New York: Harper and Row.

Seibold, D., S. M. Rossi, C. Bertotti, S. Soprych, and L. McQuillan. 1987. "Volunteer Involvement in a Hospice Program." *American Journal of Hospice Care* 4 (3): 44–55.

Seplowin, U. M., and E. Seravalli. 1983. "The Hospice: Its Changes through Time." In *Hospice: U.S.A.*, edited by A. Kutscher et al. New York: Columbia University Press.

Shanis, H. 1985. "Impact of Medicare Certification on the Hospice Movement." *Death Studies* 9: 5–6.

Sheehan, C. 1987. "The Medical Model of Hospice Care: Why It Cannot Work in America." *American Journal of Hospice Care* 4 (2): 5–6.

Sherman, L. and W. Finn. 1987. "Ethical Dilemmas Imposed by the Medicare Hospice Regulations." *New York State Journal of Medicine* (July): 379–380.

Siebold, C. 1987. "The Hospice Movement: An Historical Analysis." Ph.D diss., Wurzweiler School of Social Work.

Siebold, C., and J. Bucher. 1990. "Access to Rural Hospice Care." Unpublished paper.

Siegel, R. 1982. "A Family Centered Program of Neonatal Intensive Care." *Health and Social Work* 7: 50–58.

Sikorska, E. 1991. "The Hospice Movement in England." *Death Studies* 15 (3): 309–16.

Silver, S. 1980. "Regulations and Certification." In *A Hospice Handbook: A New Way to Care for Dying*, edited by M. Hamilton and H. Reid. Grand Rapids, Mich.: William B. Eerdmans Publishing Co.

Silver, S. 1985. "Hospice Handbook: A Guide for Managers and Planners." *American Journal of Hospice Care* 2 (6): 10.

Silverman, P. R. 1986. *Widow to Widow*. New York: Spring Publishing Co.

Simson, S., and L. B. Wilson. 1986. "Strategies For Success" *Hospice Journal* 2 (2): 19–39.

Smith, D. H., and J. A. Granbois. 1982. "The American Way of Hospice." *Hastings Center Report* 12 (2): 8–10.

Snow, D. A., and R. D. Benford. 1988. "Ideology, Frame Resonance, and Participant Mobilization." In *International Social Movement Research*, edited by B.
Klandersmans et al. Greenwich, Conn.: JAI Press.

Spector, M., and J. I. Kitsuse. 1987. *Constructing Social Problems*. New York:
Aldine DeGruyter.

Spiegel, A. 1983. *Home Health Care: Home Birthing to Hospice*. Owing Mills,
Md.: National Health Publishing.

Spillane, E. 1979. "The Analysis of Catholic Sponsored Hospices." *Hospital
Progress* 60: 46–50.

Staggenborg, S. 1989. "Organizational and Environmental Influences on the
Development of the Pro-choice Movement." *Social Forces* 68 (1): 204–40.

Starr, P. 1982. *The Social Transformation of Medicine*. New York: Basic Books.

Steinfels, P., and R. M. Veatch, eds. 1975. *The Hastings Center Report*. New
York: Harper and Row.

Stoddard, S. 1978. *The Hospice Movement: A Better Way of Caring for the Dying*.
New York: Vintage Books.

_____. 1990. "Hospice: Approaching the 21st Century." *American Journal of
Hospice and Palliative Care* 7 (2): 27–30.

Strauss, A. 1975. *Chronic Illness and the Quality of Life*. Saint Louis: C. V. Mosby
Co.

Strauss, A., and J. Corbin. 1988. *Unending Work and Care: Managing Chronic
Illness at Home*. San Francisco: Josey Bass Publishers.

Sudnow, D. 1967. *Passing On: The Social Organization of Dying*. Englewood
Cliffs, N.J.: Prentice-Hall.

Tames, S. 1986. "The Future of Hospice Care." *Medicine and Health: Perspectives*. Washington, D.C.: McGraw-Hill.

Tehan, C. 1985. "Has Success Spoiled Hospice?" *Hastings Center Report* 15 (5):
10–13.

Tenney, R. 1988. "A Brief History of American Health Care." *American Journal
of Hospice* 5 (3): 9–13.

Tischler, L. H. 1990. "Design as Healer: Boston AIDS Hospice." *Metropolitan
Home*, September, 62.

Titmuss, R. M. 1969. *Essays on "The Welfare State."* Boston: Beacon Press.

Torrens, P. R. 1985. *Hospice Programs and Public Policy*. Chicago, Ill.: American
Hospital Publishers.

Touhey, J. F. 1989. *Caring for Persons with AIDS and Cancer*. Saint Louis:
Catholic Health Association of the United States.

Trent, B. 1988. "A Place for Living, a Place for Dying." *Canadian Medical Association Journal* 139 (9): 889–93.

Twycross, R. 1990. "Viewpoint: Assisted Death, a Reply." *Lancet* 336: 796–98.

Ufema, J. K. 1989. "Is This Hospice?" *American Journal of Hospice Care* 6 (1): 71.

Vachon, M. 1986. "Myths and Realities in Palliative and Hospice Care." *Hospice Journal* 2 (1): 63–79.

Veatch, R. M. 1988. "Justice and the Economics of Terminal Illness." *Hastings Center Report* 18: 34–40.

Wakefield, D., J. P. Curry, and S. E. Kieffer. 1987. "Organizational and Operational Characteristics of Hospice Programs in Iowa." *American Journal of Hospice Care* 4 (3): 35–42.

Wald, F. 1989. "The Widening Scope of Spiritual Care." *American Journal of Hospice Care* 6 (4): 40–43.

Wald, F., Z. Foster, and H. Wald. 1980. "The Hospice Movement as a Health Care Reform." *Nursing Outlook*, March, 173–78.

Wald, H. J. 1983. "The Hospice Community as Reform." In *Hospice: USA*, edited by A. Kutscher et al. New York: Columbia University Press.

Wallace, W. 1990. "Clinical Issues Which Affect Care." *American Journal of Hospice and Palliative Care* 7 (3): 13–16.

Walsh, E. J. 1978. "Mobilization Theory vis-à-vis a Mobilization Process." In *Research in Social Movements, Conflicts and Change*, edited by L. Kriesberg. Greenwich, Conn.: JAI Press.

_____. 1981. "Resource Mobilization and Citizen Protest in Communities around Three Mile Island." *Social Problems* 29 (1): 1–21.

Wanzer, S. H., D. D. Federman, S. J. Adelstein, et al. 1989. "The Physician's Responsibility toward Hopelessly Ill Patients: A Second Look." *New England Journal of Medicine* 320 (13): 844–49.

Wass, H. 1979. *Dying: Facing the Facts*. Washington, D.C.: Hemisphere Publishing Corp.

Waugh, E. 1948. *The Loved One*. Boston: Little, Brown and Co.

Weeks, D. 1989. "Death Education: For Aspiring Physicians, Teachers, and Funeral Directors." *Death Studies* 13 (1): 17–24.

Weir, R. 1986. *Ethical Issues in Death and Dying*. New York: Columbia University Press.

Wilkinson, H. J. 1986. "Assessment of Patients Satisfaction of Hospice: A Review and Investigation." *Hospice Journal* 2 (4): 69–94.

Wilkinson, H. J., D. MacDonald, L. Pelz. 1990. "An Assessment of New York Hospice Programs." *American Journal of Hospice and Palliative Care* 7 (4): 31–38.

Williams, R. W. 1989. "Another Look at Hospice in America." *American Journal of Hospice Care* 6 (5): 15–16.

_____. 1990. "Which Came First: The Hospice or the Funding?" *American Journal of Hospice and Palliative Care* 7 (4): 21–26.

Wilson, D. C. 1982. "The Viability of Pediatric Hospices: A Case Study." *Death Education* 6: 205–12.

Wilson, D. C., T. Ajemian, and B. M. Mount. 1978. "Montreal 1975: The Royal Victoria Hospital Palliative Care Service." In *The Hospice Movement*, edited by G. W. Davidson. Washington, D.C.: Hemisphere Publishing Corp.

Wylie, N. A. 1978. "Halifax 1976: Victorial General Hospital." In *The Hospice Movement*, edited by G. W. Davidson. Washington, D.C.: Hemisphere Publishing Corp.

Yancey, D., and H. A. Greger. 1990. "Determinants of Grief Resolution in Cancer Death." *Journal of Palliative Care* 6 (4): 24–34.

Zimmer, J. G., J. A. Groth, J. McCusker. 1984. "Effects of a Physician-led Home Care Team on Terminal Care." *Journal of American Geriatric Society* 32 (4): 288–92.

Zimmerman, J. M. 1981. *Hospice: Complete Care for the Terminally Ill.* Baltimore: Urban and Scharzenberg.

Zola, I. K. 1978. "Medicine as an Institution of Social Control: The Medicalizing of a Society." In *Basic Readings in Medical Sociology*, edited by D. Tuckett and J. M. Kurfert. London: Tavistock Publications.

# Index

# The Author

Cathy Siebold, D.S.W., L.C.S.W., received her doctorate from Yeshiva University and her master's degree from New York University. She currently teaches at the University of Southern Maine in the Department of Social Work and previously taught at Penn State University. Dr. Siebold has spent most of her career as a psychotherapist and has worked extensively with the terminally ill and their survivors. Her articles have appeared in *Clinical Social Work* and *Smith College Studies in Social Work*.